Aromatherapy
For
Common Illnesses

A Beginner's Guide
to Mixing Essential Oils

Kath Hoskisson-Craven©

Published in the United Kingdom

Content Copywrite © Kathryn Hoskisson-Craven 2017

Illustrations Copywrite © Kathryn Hoskisson-Craven 2017

A CIP record of this book is available from the British Library

First Printed August 2017

Disclaimer: This book is not a substitute for proper medical advice. It is recommended that a firm diagnosis by a medical practitioner has been made before treatment. The author, editor, and publisher do not claim that aromatherapy can heal any medical conditions.

Acknowledgements

There are so many people that I have to thank, for their support and advice, without which I would never have written this book.

Firstly I have to thank my Copywriter, Anne-Marie Emerson McDonald, of Emerson Editing (www.emersonediting.com), who calmly and efficiently guided me through the editing of this book. I could not have done this without her.

Then I would like to acknowledge a whole bunch of gorgeous goddesses who came to help me in my hour of need. They read through my drafts and gave me very good advice on how to make it better. Their support made me carry on even when I thought I couldn't do it. So thanks to Katie Grant, Rebecca Campbell, Kelly Morgan, Nikki Morgan, and Kristen Wruck Hammer; you truly are Unicorn Goddesses.

Finally I need to express my gratitude to my loving husband Andy, who has tolerated my absences whilst I type, put up with my books and oils lying all over the place, and has supported me throughout this experience.

Foreword

When I was a child I would play with making perfumes and scents from the flowers in springtime. I would bury my head in the cherry blossom, roses and herbs that smelt so good, and try to make the scent stay long after I had collected the petals that had fallen to the floor. Obviously the scent never stayed for long as the flowers wilted and died.

Then in my teenage years I was introduced to Lavender to use on my spots, and tea tree from Australia to use on cuts and bruises. I was fascinated with the claims that these oils could help people heal just by putting them on your skin. It was interesting to see Tea Tree candles and oils being burnt in rooms in the hospital where I first worked as a nurse, especially in rooms where MRSA was prevalent. I wanted to know how and why they seemed to help in getting people better. It couldn't possibly just be the medication they were on....

So in my early twenties I looked further into essential oils and their healing properties, educating myself and using oils to treat everyday problems that arose. I would take a first aid kit of essential oils with me when I travelled, and treat family and friends where I could. This eventually led me to take my Aromatherapy qualification.

However, throughout all my years of working with oils I had never found a single book that would give me an easy method of combining the oils to help with more than issue at a time.

Yes there were recipes to follow for a problem, but that only treated one issue at a time. Yes there were books that listed the oils and told you what they were useful for, but you had to trawl through the book to find all the oils you were looking for and then see if they actually smelt good together. Then there were tables that listed all the oils for one issue but didn't tell you if they were good together.

I felt that there had to be a better way.

So five years after I started researching this book I have finally written a definitive guide to treating common illnesses; that can combine oils to treat not just one but two or three at the same time, and that you can check simply and quickly to see if the oils should work together well. Illnesses often have more than one symptom and this book will show you how to treat these using just one mix. It will also help you choose the right method of using the oils to its best advantage, and give you tips on the right mix, use and what to avoid.

It's been a long journey, of learning and experience to get this book to the point it is at now; ready for you the reader to try your own hand at mixing oils. There is no wrong or right way, so don't worry about trying a mix and finding it smells awful. This book is about experimenting to find your own beautiful scents like I did as a child, with my head in a bucket of cherry blossom.

Kath xx

Table of Contents

What is aromatherapy and how does it work?

Aromatherapy, like herbalism, has been around for thousands of years.

The earliest records show that gums from trees were used for ailments and perfumes, and were prized for their healing abilities. Frankincense and myrrh were as precious as gold in some cultures. In a world without human-made medicine it was to plants and herbs that people turned, not only using them in cooking and physical healing but also for rituals and ceremonies.

The smell, aroma, and probably microscopic molecules of certain plant extracts were known to influence the brain and send people into trances, calm them or excite them for battle.

Over the years more has become known about the effects of essential oils on the person, how to get the best oil from the plant, and the best methods of getting them into the body. This is now known as aromatherapy.

The scent of essential oils has an immediate effect on our bodies. When we breathe in the smell, the cells in our nose are stimulated which affects the emotional centre of the brain.

This area of the brain is linked to memory, breathing, blood circulation and the regulation of hormone production levels in the body.

It is the properties of the oils, including the fragrance and its effects, which determine how these systems of the body are affected.

This is the emotional effect of the oils, helping to calm the nerves and give a sense of healthy balance between body and mind.

Scientists have now broken down essential oils into their chemical components, and their action is well documented.

When essential oils make contact with the skin through massage, in a bath, or even when we breathe, the smell of the oils is inhaled and the microscopic molecules are also absorbed by the skin.

They enter the tissues of the body through hair follicles, sweat glands or the mucous membranes of the mouth. They go into the bloodstream where they make their way to our organs and other systems of the body.

Once inside they have many valuable effects such as:

Strengthening and stimulating the immune system

Speeding up digestion and the elimination of toxins

Helping new cell growth and stimulating the healing process

Therefore, essential oils, when used correctly, enable the body to heal itself.

However, aromatherapy is not meant to be a replacement for medical care but can be used as complementary to it. It can, in some cases, offer an alternative to over-the-counter medications or even prescription medications.

Essential oils can be extremely good at treating wounds, cuts, bruises, any area that is inflamed or stiff, acne and spots and many other common ailments that you may have.

It can also help with stress, anxiety, tiredness and fatigue.

However, do not think that aromatherapy alone will 'cure' you. It has to be used along with other mainstream treatments to be beneficial.

The old saying that 'you have to get worse to get better' is actually true in aromatherapy as many people experience what is known as a 'healing crisis' for several days after using them.

This healing crisis is the body's way of cleansing and healing itself, ultimately becoming stronger. It is often associated with producing more antibodies to fight the illness or infection. The symptoms can often be rather unpleasant and can be mistaken for an illness or sickness such as a feeling of having a cold or flu. Joints may ache and original symptoms may appear to become worse. However, it is simply your body overcoming this ill health, becoming healthier and stronger. It will pass within a few days.

If symptoms remain after five days then it possible that it is an actual illness and medical attention should be sought. It has been known that a healing crisis can trigger another illness to overcome the original one, such as getting tonsillitis as the body gets rid of its toxins. This is completely normal and will pass.

So what are essential oils?

Essential oils used in aromatherapy are derived from the leaves, stems, roots, bark or flowers of a plant. They are liquids which can be mixed with a carrier oil to make them go further, or with other essential oils to make a rich aromatic beneficial 'potion' to use.

Essential oils are not fragrance oils, which are like perfume oils and have synthetic substances in them, making them completely useless for therapeutic purposes.

Essential oils are extracted from the plants in various ways such as steam distillation, cold or hot pressed, or water distillation. Most, but not all, result in a clear liquid.

All essential oils are made up of chemical compounds. Some have similar chemical compounds, as the plant is in the same 'family' of other plants; while others can be unique. These chemical compounds are the components that provide the healing that oils are renowned for. These are absorbed into your blood stream where they act like chemicals and help the issue you are treating.

It would be too complicated to list all the chemical compounds for each oil on the bottle label and it would probably not be any help to you anyway. Therefore, books like this are written to help you decide which oils are best to use for your issue.

How essential oils are made.

There are three main methods for getting oils from plant material. Each is used to produce a specific type of essential oil.

<u>Expression</u>

The expression method is only used for citrus fruits as these oils are very close to the surface of the peel. This means they can be extracted easily by squeezing or scarification (where the skin is punctured with very fine needles to let out the oil).

The oil is soaked up with a sponge which is then processed to get the essential oil out and bottled up.

<u>Distillation</u>

This process involves a lot of heat. The plant material being used is heated up until it produces a vapour.

Then this vapour is cooled rapidly and becomes a liquid.

Steam distillation uses steam under pressure to get the oil out quickly. The steam is then separated from the oil which is heavier than water when cooled. This method is very good for delicate oils which may be damaged by heat.

Water distillation is a much slower method, where the plant material is covered in water and heated in a vacuum-sealed container. The resulting water is separated from the oil in a variety of ways.

<u>Solvent extraction</u>

Any plant part which is too delicate to be subjected to heat, or only has a small amount of essential oil in it, can go through solvent extraction as a gentler method.

This method uses a hydrocarbon solvent rather than water, as the solvent evaporates at a lower temperature than water. However, the resulting oil, resin or concrete (a waxy harder substance) can still contain fragments of the solvent and may have to go through another process to purify it.

Nowadays, experiments are being carried out on a different process that produces high quality oils without contamination. This is called hypercritical carbon dioxide and is a very expensive method of extraction.

Oils that are produced in this manner tend to be expensive themselves or difficult to obtain.

The concretes that are obtained cannot be used as essential oils straight away and have to go through another process of solvent extraction -- except this time either alcohol or liquid carbon dioxide is used rather than hydrocarbon substances.

This process produces something called an 'absolute'.

If the absolute has been made with alcohol it needs to be further purified to get rid of any leftover alcohol, and in most cases this cannot be achieved. Any oil that still contains alcohol is not really suitable for use in aromatherapy.

Therefore, the oil made by liquid carbon dioxide is the purer of the two and can be used. Check the label carefully of any absolute to ensure there is no alcohol present.

In both methods the resulting substance can be thicker than most essential oils.

Aromatherapy 'notes'

Aromatherapy divides oils up according to their 'notes', or ability to evaporate when exposed to air. There are top notes, middle notes, and base or bottom notes. All three notes should be blended together to make a balanced scent.

Top notes are the most volatile and lose their smell very quickly - between one and two hours after applying. They are light and fresh, usually made from flowers and leaves including flowering herbs. They are uplifting and stimulating oils. Top notes work very quickly and start the healing process off.

Middle notes lose their smell between two and four hours after application. They are usually made from spices and herbs using the whole plant and tend to balance the smells of top and base notes.

Base or bottom notes keep their smell the longest, and some can even last for days. They are heavy and rich, made from the gums and resins of trees, and are the last to be smelt. Base notes work deeply to treat underlying chronic illness or problems, carrying on the healing process from the top notes.

Perfumery notes

Top	Middle	Base
Basil	Black Pepper	Benzoin
Bergamot	Carrot Seed	Cedarwood
Cajuput	Chamomile	Cinnamon
Clary Sage (also middle)	German Chamomile	Frankincense
Eucalyptus	Roman	Ginger
Grapefruit	Clary Sage (also top)	Jasmine
Lemon		Myrrh
Lemongrass	Cypress	Neroli
		Patchouli

Top	Middle	Base
Lime	Geranium	Rose
Mandarin	Juniper	Sandalwood
May Chang (Litsea Cubeba)	Lavender	Valerian
Niaouli	Marjoram	Vetiver
Orange	Melissa	Ylang Ylang (Also middle)
Peppermint (also middle)	Parsley	
Petitgrain	Peppermint (also top)	
Tea Tree	Pine (Scotch)	
Thyme	Rosemary	
Verbena	Spearmint	
	Sweet Fennel	
	Ylang Ylang (Also base)	

Oils to avoid

Because of the chemical properties and the way they work on the body, in some cases people should avoid certain oils. This is very important and is included in the form at the back of this book.

Condition	Oils to avoid
Diabetes	Angelica
Epilepsy	Fennel Rosemary
Hypertension / high blood pressure	Rosemary Clary Sage Thyme (any kind)

Condition	Oils to avoid
Pregnancy: avoid at any time	Basil Clary Sage Jasmine Juniper Peppermint Rosemary Thyme
Pregnancy: avoid in first trimester, then diluted to 1-2% :	Lavender Rose Geranium Chamomile
Sensitive skin	Basil Bergamot Black Pepper Eucalyptus Geranium German Chamomile Ginger Jasmine Lemon Lemongrass Neroli Peppermint Chamomile Roman Tea Tree Valerian

If you have sensitive skin you should conduct a skin test on a small area on the inside of your wrist, and leave for 24 hours. If there is any irritation, swelling or redness do not use this oil.

The following oils should not be used in either steam inhalation or in the bath:

Frankincense / Citrus oils

The following oils should not be used for longer than two weeks at a time:

Juniper

Cinnamon

Valerian

Eucalyptus

The following oils should never be used as they can cause poisoning and are extremely toxic:

Aniseed	Red Thyme
Arnica	Rue
Bitter Fennel	Sassafras
Bitter Orange	Savoury
Cedar	Tansy
Common Sage	Wintergreen
Mugwort	Wormwood
Pine (dwarf)	

Carrier oils

Most essential oils have to be diluted in another oil before applying to the skin. This other oil is known as a carrier oil.

These carrier oils are always vegetable in origin, mostly from the fatty part of the plant such nuts or seeds, so care must be taken in choosing a carrier oil if you or your client are allergic to nuts.

Carrier oils will not evaporate, and can have therapeutic values in their own right.

They are all absorbed into the skin easily and the best ones are cold pressed and unrefined.

Different carrier oils have different properties and aromas, and it is important to choose one specific to your needs.

<u>Sweet almond oil</u>

This is the most common carrier oil in aromatherapy.

It is pale yellow in colour, with practically no odour to interfere with the smell of the essential oils used. It is rich in minerals and vitamins with some protein as well.

Sweet almond oil is great for dry, sensitive or irritated skin, which is one of the reasons it is so popular. It is also softening and nourishing, making it excellent for massage.

<u>Apricot kernel oil</u>

This is a darker yellow in colour, yet has a light silky feel to it. It is absorbed quickly into the skin, making it excellent for small massage areas such as the face.

Apricot kernel oil is suitable for mature, dry, sensitive or irritated skin due to its vitamin and mineral content.

Avocado oil

Some people are put off using this lovely nutty-smelling oil because of its deep green colour. It is quite viscous and deeply penetrating and should be used in combination with other lighter oils in a 25:75% mix.

Being very rich and nutritious, avocado oil is very good for skin that needs nourishment, is dry, dehydrated or mature. It is also good for the treatment of eczema.

Calendula oil

This is an infused oil, meaning that the oily parts of the plant have been infused in a base oil of some kind, putting all of the goodness into that actual oil.

Calendula oil is brilliant for its healing properties as it aids tissue regeneration, so it can be used for rashes, cracked skin, bruises and burns.

Carrot oil

This oil is also an infused oil made from the root of the carrot plant. It should not be confused with carrot seed oil; these oils are made from two completely different parts of the plant.

Carrot oil is orange in colour, and like the plant itself, is rich in beta-carotene and vitamins. This combination is great for aging skin, or dry, itchy or inflamed skin.

However, due to its colour and richness it is best used diluted with a light carrier oil in a 10% dilution (i.e. 10ml carrot oil plus 90ml other base oil such as sweet almond).

Coconut oil

Reminiscent of tropical days on the beach, coconut oil is solid at room temperature, and can be used in creams or on the hair.

There are too many benefits of good quality 100% virgin coconut oil to mention here, but information is readily available elsewhere.

Evening primrose oil

Lots of people take evening primrose oil supplements as part of their daily routine, but this golden yellow oil is also fabulous as a moisturizing base for other essential oils.

It should be used sparingly as it is expensive, so use it in a 20% mix with another carrier oil.

Evening primrose oil is good for dry, aging skin, stress and psoriasis.

Grapeseed oil

This oil is only available as a refined oil but it is popular with Aromatherapists because of its fine, easily absorbed texture.

It is pale green and is an excellent mixer for other heavier oils that need diluting before use such as evening primrose, or carrot oil as mentioned above.

Hazelnut oil

Hazelnut oil has a sweet nutty smell that compliments its pale yellow colour. It is easily absorbed into the skin as it is very light in texture and is also mildly astringent. This makes it great for oily or inflamed skin.

If the smell is too much for you, you can mix it in with another carrier oil to reduce the nutty aroma.

Jojoba oil

This is actually not an oil at all but a liquid wax, yet it acts like any other carrier oil.

Jojoba is light, deeply penetrating and moisturising, and its chemical makeup is very similar to the substance sebum in our skin, making it excellent for any skin type.

Aromatherapists like jojoba because it can be used on just about anyone; however, it can be expensive.

Rosehip seed oil

Rosehip seed oil can vary in colour from pale yellow to rich orange and has good tissue regeneration properties. It is a popular oil for helping to reduce the signs of aging, making it suited to mature, dry and sun-damaged skins.

It is very rich, so is best used in a 20% dilution with another carrier oil.

Methods of using oils to their best advantage

<u>Inhalation</u>

Inhaling essential oils can help with a variety of ailments and conditions. Oils can be inhaled using steam, or even in an oil burner in the room.

Inhaling provides both mental and physical benefits as the aroma stimulates brain activity. Taking it into the lungs allows the different chemical compounds to pass into the blood stream, providing the therapeutic benefits.

To inhale using steam inhalation place boiling water into a bowl, and then place between 6-8 drops of the oil or oil mix straight into the bowl. Lean over the bowl and inhale deeply. You can cover your head with a towel if you want to (it makes a great facial steam too).

Be aware that some oils will tickle the back of your throat or feel as though they are burning you at first. If you find this is the case either stop using them, or move further away from the bowl.

<u>Applying oils to the skin</u>

When essential oils are applied to the skin they are absorbed directly into the epidermis and your bloodstream. The epidermis is the layers that make up the skin on our body. Therefore, applying oils directly to the area affected can help healing.

Unless stated otherwise in this book, essential oils should be diluted with a carrier oil before applying. These are discussed later on in this book.

Using massage as a medium to get the oils into the skin and blood stream can help with stress and anxiety so can be very calming. Reducing stress can help with dis-ease in the body and thus speed up the healing process.

Add around 10 drops of the oil mix to 30ml of carrier oil or 3-5 drops per 5ml. Mix well. This diluted oil can be poured onto the hand and then applied to the body.

Do not use near the genital area or eyes as some oils can sting badly.

<u>Tissue inhalation</u>

Sometimes you just need a quick pick-me-up and can't get to a steam inhaler. This is when drops of essential oil on a tissue can help.

Place between two and four drops of your chosen oil onto a tissue and hold this near your nose and inhale (through your nose of course). It is best to use only one oil at a time with this method.

The oil will be inhaled and taken into your blood stream via the delicate membranes in your nasal cavity.

If it's your first time using a particular oil in this way make sure that you use only one drop to start with, to test for any adverse reaction or sensitivity.

<u>Room diffuser (oil burner)</u>

Sometimes it is not relevant to use either steam inhalation or a tissue. This may be because the person is too ill, too young or too old or has a particular sensitivity.

Whatever the reason, you can still get the oils to work in your favour.

You can add 8–12 drops of your oil mix (with a carrier oil to make it go further) to either a room oil burner, or use the steam inhalation method and instead of putting your face over it, let the steam diffuse into the room.

This is useful for an oil that you are sensitive to or that is not recommended for direct inhalation.

It will work the same way, but it will just take longer to work.

<u>Baths</u>

There is a lot of debate on how to get oils to work in water, so I have included several ways. Experiment to find out which way suits you best.

In all cases use around 10 drops of essential oil or essential oil mixture in 30ml of carrier oil or other liquid as stated below.

If oil is put straight into a bath it will float on the top of the water. You can mix it as well as you can but some will still remain on top.

Therefore, a lot of the oil will make it onto your skin as you get out of the bath. If it's only just got onto your skin you need to leave it there without towelling it off straight away. Try just patting your skin dry.

You can use Epsom salts to make a mix with your oil and this will dissolve in the warm water allowing the oils to dissipate into it. However, some of the oil will just float to the surface again. But using Epsom salts is in itself beneficial in a bath, so this method may work for you.

Believe it or not oils will mix well with either alcohol or milk.

Use a cheap vodka which does not smell or have any particular additives in it and add the oils directly to 30mls of it. Blend well and then add to the bath, making sure you mix it around in the water.

Do not use whisky, beer, cider or wine -- you may consume these at your own risk instead.

Any type of milk will allow the oils to be mixed in before adding to the bath. Use around 30ml of milk and swish this (with the oils mixed in) into the bath water before immersing. If milk was good enough for Cleopatra then it's good enough for us.

Using alcohol or milk is an excellent way of getting the oils to disperse in the bath water rather than stay on the surface.

<u>Sitz baths</u>

Sometimes we need to just bathe the genital area rather than the whole body, or we need to get the oils into this area on a regular basis.

So rather than having to run a whole bath, we can use a Sitz bath instead.

A Sitz bath is basically a bath that is filled only 3-4 inches high with water, which can then be sat in. It's a version of a bidet for those people who don't have one.

The oils can be added directly to the water as it doesn't matter if the oils sit on the surface. If you do not want to sit down, you can kneel in the water and splash the water onto the area instead. Either way the oils will reach the places you want them to. Make sure the water is warm and not too hot.

Add 6-10 drops of the chosen oil (or a mixture) to the Sitz bath and mix well before getting in.

<u>Cold compress</u>

A cold compress is basically a cold wet cloth that is soaked in a mixture of the oils and water and placed on the affected area.

Add around 5-6 drops of your oil or oil mix to a bowl of cold water. This oil will lie on the surface of the water.

Soak a clean cloth or facecloth as close to the surface of the water as possible to get the oils on to it, then wring out into the bowl and place on the area needed. You can cover the cloth with another towel or bandage to keep in place.

Re-soak the cloth as soon as it becomes warm again – check after every five minutes.

<u>Hot compress</u>

A hot compress is made by adding around 5-6 drops of your oil or oil mix into a basin of hot (not boiling) water. Soak a facecloth or clean cloth in this as close to the surface as possible to collect as much oil as you can, wring slightly to remove excess water and place on the affected area. Re-soak the cloth as soon as it becomes cold.

If the water goes cold, you can reheat it in the microwave (don't boil it and be aware that the smell and taste of the oils can transfer to the microwave so wash the oven before the next use); or you could add more hot water to it, allowing it to settle (and bring the oils back to the surface) before you soak the cloth again.

<u>Hair care</u>

You can either add a few drops of the oil to the final rinse or a cheap gentle shampoo, or make an alcohol based hair rub by adding around 1 teaspoon of the oil or oil mix to around 100ml of vodka.

Wash the hair with this and then, if required by the issue being treated, use a carrier oil with oils in it and leave on for a couple of hours or even overnight. (Wrap your hair in a towel during this time). The hair can then be washed as normal again.

<u>Gargles</u>

Using a gargle can help with mouth or throat issues; however, it is very important not to swallow the solution.

To make a gargle place 1-2 drops of the oil or oil mix into a glass of warm water and mix thoroughly.

Gargle for up to 30 seconds and then spit out.

Alternatively use virgin coconut oil (1 tablespoon) melted for a couple of seconds in the microwave and add the essential oils to this. Use like mouthwash by swooshing around the mouth and gargle for 30 seconds to two minutes and then spit out into a jar.

Coconut oil should never be put down the sink as it solidifies as soon as it gets cold and could potentially block your pipes!

<u>Foot baths</u>

Fill a bowl or foot spa with enough hot/warm water to cover the feet, and add 6-8 drops of essential oil or oil mix to it. Mix thoroughly and place feet into the solution for 10-20 minutes. Pat dry afterwards.

Part One

Using the Book

How to use this book

For the purposes of this book it doesn't matter how the oil is taken from the plant, or the medicinal / chemical properties that make up the plant. There are other books that can describe these in more detail if required.

This book is intended to help you mix the right oils together to treat common ailments at home. This could be just one illness or up to three at a time.

Forty-six of the most common oils are used, but in order to have a basic kit, it is recommended that you have access to the following oils:

Benzoin

Bergamot

Cedarwood

Chamomile

Cinnamon

Clary Sage

Cypress

Geranium

Lavender

Lemon

Myrrh

Rosemary

Tea Tree

These can also be used as an emergency kit.

Some illnesses are common and their symptoms are known to most people without having to go to a doctor, but others are more serious and should only be treated after a definite diagnosis from a medical practitioner.

It is important that you are certain of the illness or condition before treating yourself or others with aromatherapy.

Additionally, and very importantly, if you are already taking homeopathy tablets then aromatherapy must be avoided completely. The chemicals in the oils will negate the effects of the homeopathy.

Please note: All the oils which could cause a reaction to sensitive skin, or have to be avoided in certain conditions such as pregnancy, epilepsy or high blood pressure, are indicated in every table in the conditions section with a *. Please check the 'oils to avoid' section when you want to use any oil with this symbol next to it.

Mixing oils

To mix oils together, always use a combination of top, middle and bottom notes wherever possible.

Because essential oils evaporate and lose their potency over different lengths of time, you should mix them in proper proportions according to the following formula:

2 drops of top

7 drops of middle

1 drop of base

Base oils can be very overpowering, so need to be used sparingly, whereas middle oils are the glue which hold the top and base together. Therefore, it makes sense to use more middle oil and less of the other two.

Where oils can be classed between two of the categories they are very useful in bringing a mix together.

Getting Started

There are 59 different conditions listed in this book, with oils that help treat the condition listed in their perfumery notes (top, middle or bottom).

The tables for each condition look like this example:

Oils		
Top	**Middle**	**Base**
Bergamot	Chamomile	Ylang Ylang
Eucalyptus	Geranium	
Lemon	Lavender	

The idea of this book is to try and treat all your symptoms and/or conditions in one go, by finding all the oils that are common to those symptoms and/or conditions.

To do this you need to complete four easy stages:

<u>Step one</u>:

Print off / copy the form at the end of this book, then go through this book and look up your first condition, illness or symptom that you want to treat.

Use the form and tick off all the oils that are listed for that condition or symptom.

Now look up the second condition, illness, or symptom and do the same. You can repeat this for everything you wish to treat at once. Aromatherapists tend to focus on the top three issues you have at the time and this is how the form is set out, but you could try more if you wish.

Eventually you will end up with a list that like this:

| Note | Condition | | | Note | Condition | | | Note | Condition | | |
| Top | 1 | 2 | 3 | Middle | 1 | 2 | 3 | Base | 1 | 2 | 3 |
	Cold	Cough	Catarrh		Cold	Cough	Catarrh		Cold	Cough	Catarrh
Basil	√		√	Black Pepper	√	√	√	Benzoin	√	√	√
Bergamot	√		√	Carrot Seed		√		Cedarwood	√	√	√
Cajuput	√			Chamomile			√	Cinnamon		√	
Clary Sage		√		Clary Sage		√		Frankincense	√		
Eucalyptus	√	√	√	Cypress		√		Ginger	√	√	√
Grapefruit	√			Geranium	√			Jasmine		√	√
Lemon	√	√	√	Juniper	√	√	√	Myrrh	√	√	√
Lime				Lavender	√	√		Neroli		√	√
Lemongrass		√		Marjoram	√		√	Patchouli			
Litsea cubeba	√	√		Melissa	√	√	√	Rose			
Mandarin				Peppermint	√	√	√	Sandalwood		√	
Niaouli	√	√	√	Pine (Scotch)	√	√	√	Valerian		√	√
Orange				Rosemary	√	√	√	Vetiver			
Peppermint	√	√	√	Sweet Fennel				Ylang Ylang			
Petitgrain	√										
Tea Tree		√	√								
Thyme		√									
Verbena											

<u>Step two:</u>

Once you have looked up all ailments you wish to treat (up to three at any one time), choose one oil from the top notes, one from the middle notes, and one from the base which is common to all three conditions.

In the chart above there are lots of oils that cover all three conditions:

Oils		
Top	**Middle**	**Base**
Eucalyptus	Black Pepper	Benzoin
Lemon	Juniper	Cedarwood
Niaouli	Melissa	Frankincense
Peppermint	Peppermint	Ginger
Thyme	Pine (Scotch)	Myrrh
	Rosemary	

Now check to see if the oils you have chosen are compatible with each other by using the oil compatibility charts in appendix 1.

In my example I can deduce several options:

Option 1: Lemon, Melissa, Benzoin

Option 2: Eucalyptus, Pine (Scotch), Frankincense

Option 3: Lemon, Juniper, Cedarwood

<u>Step three:</u>

Check out the Oil Compatibility Charts in Appendix One. These will tell you if the oils you have chosen will mix well together. If not try changing the mix until you have one that may be compatible.

Test the combined smell by dropping one drop of each oil onto a separate cotton bud and holding together to smell. If the scent is agreeable then use these oils in the following quantities:

2 drops of top oil

7 drops of middle oil

1 drops of base oil

This becomes a synergy mix and is very powerful. If you need more, just double the quantities.

If a condition only has one or two oils listed ensure one of these is included in your mix. This should also be the case where there may be only one note shown.

If you are using the oils just for massage purposes, then you can use the whole synergy mix combined with 10-30 ml of your preferred carrier oil.

<u>Step four:</u>

Lastly see what (if any) method of use is suggested by each condition and use the most common one. If there isn't a method suggested then use the one you feel most comfortable with. This will usually be massage over the area affected.

For example, in the conditions used in the above example (cold, cough and catarrh), there are several methods of use listed - steam inhalation, bath and massage. In this instance I would choose steam inhalation and massaging across the throat, neck and chest.

Even if there were no methods listed I would consider the condition and decide on the best method based on my common sense. Anything sore would be massage based, and anything internal would be a different method.

Please note: In some cases it is not advisable to treat all the conditions in one go due to the nature of the primary issue. For instance, head lice should be treated on its own as the method of application is directly onto the head and hair. Check the description of the condition and suggested methods of using the oils, and use common sense in these instances

.

Part Two

The Conditions

Conditions

A	B
Abscesses	Bleeding Gums
Acne	Blocked Nose
Anxiety	Blood Pressure – High
Arthritis	Blood Pressure – Low
Asthma	
Athletes Foot	

C	D
Catarrh	Depression
Cold Sores / Herpes	Dermatitis / Eczema
Colds	Diarrhoea
Constipation	
Coughs – general	
Cracked dry skin / lips	
Cramp	
Cuts	
Cystitis	

E	F
Earache	Flatulence
	Flu
	Fluid Retention / Oedema)

G	H
Gastroenteritis	Haemorrhoids
Gout	Headaches
	Heartburn
	High Temperature (Fever)

I	**L**
Indigestion (Dyspepsia)	Laryngitis
Insect Stings or Bites	
Irritable Bowel Syndrome	
M	**N**
Migraine	Nausea
Mouth Ulcers	
Muscular Aches and Pains	
P	**R**
Palpitations	Rheumatism
Premenstrual Tension /	
Premenstrual Syndrome	
S	**T**
Scars	Throat Infections
Sciatica	Tonsillitis
Sinusitis	Toothache
Sore Throat / Pharyngitis	
Spasms / Muscle cramps	
Stomach Ache	
Stiffness	
Stress	
Stretch Marks	
U	**V**
Urinary Tract Infections	Vomiting
W	
Wounds	Wrinkles

Abscesses

An abscess is a cavity that is filled with pus, that is either been caused by a foreign object such as an ingrown hair or splinter, or by a bacterial or parasite infection. If it is on the skin the area will be inflamed and may be hard to the touch. Alternatively it may have a distinctive yellow 'head' on it.

Essential oils diluted in carrier oils and used in a hot compress over the affected area, or essential oils placed in the bath, can sometimes help to relieve the symptoms. For dental abscesses, a hot compress applied to the face using Lavender and Tea Tree essential oils can sometimes help to relieve the symptoms whilst waiting to visit a dentist. The most effective oils for treating abscesses are Chamomile German, Chamomile Roman, Lavender, Tea Tree and Thyme oils.

Oils for Abscesses		
Top	**Middle**	**Base**
Bergamot*	Chamomile*	Myrrh
Clary Sage*	Clary Sage*	Rose*
Eucalyptus*	Juniper*	
Lemon*	Lavender*	
Niaouli		
Tea Tree*		

Oils for Abscesses		
Top	**Middle**	**Base**
Thyme*		

Acne

Acne is a skin rash that often affects teenagers and young adults, although older people can also have it. Acne can appear anywhere on the body but is usually more predominant on the face, chest, neck and back, where the body produces more oil.

Left untreated acne can cause quite severe scarring, but even in the short term self-confidence can be damaged.

Cosmetics can cause further irritation and should be avoided, as should scrubbing the affected areas. Gentle washing with soap and water to remove excess oil, or using specialist over-the-counter acne remedies, has more effect. In severe cases, especially in older adults, medical treatment should be sought as the issue may be unrelated to excess oil and infection may be occurring.

Oils for Acne		
Top	**Middle**	**Base**
Bergamot*	Carrot Seed	Cedarwood
Cajuput	Chamomile*	Cinnamon
		Frankincense

Oils for Acne		
Top	**Middle**	**Base**
Clary Sage*	Clary Sage*	Neroli*
Grapefruit	Geranium*	Patchouli
Lemon*	Juniper*	Rose*
Lemongrass	Lavender*	Sandalwood
Lime	Peppermint*	Vetiver
Mandarin	Rosemary*	Ylang Ylang
May Chang (Litsea Cubeba)		
Niaouli		
Peppermint*		
Petitgrain		
Tea Tree*		

Top Tip: Evening primrose and jojoba carrier oils can either be used to mix with these essential oils or used on their own. Use as a massage oil on the face.

Anxiety

Anxiety can be a normal, healthy response to certain stressful situations. However, when it is out of control or occurring for no rational reason it can become a more serious condition.

Anxiety is often described as feeling fear, worry or apprehension but it can also have physical symptoms associated with it. These may include nausea, chest pain, headaches, sweating, trembling, pale skin and palpitations.

In severe cases anxiety may be referred to as panic, which comes on suddenly and lasts for 10 minutes or more. These types of attacks generally occur after frightening events, or prolonged stress.

Panic attacks tend to have individual symptoms as well as general ones. All symptoms of normal anxiety can be experienced but are heightened due to a higher awareness of what's going on in their body. Additional symptoms can include a feeling of paralysis, impending doom, dizziness, fainting and confusion.

Severe anxiety should only be treated in conjunction with professional counselling.

Oils for Anxiety		
Top	**Middle**	**Base**
Bergamot*	Chamomile Roman*	Cedarwood
Clary Sage*	Clary Sage*	Frankincense
Verbena	Cypress	Jasmine*
	Geranium*	Neroli*
	Juniper*	Patchouli
	Lavender*	Rose*

Oils for Anxiety		
Top	**Middle**	**Base**
	Marjoram	Sandalwood
	Melissa	Ylang Ylang
	Ylang Ylang	

Arthritis

There are different types of arthritis such as osteoarthritis (the most common form), which affects the joints making them swollen, stiff and painful; and rheumatoid arthritis, which is an autoimmune disease where the body's natural defences suddenly start attacking healthy tissues.

In rheumatoid arthritis the damage caused by the disease can affect the surrounding areas as well, but is usually restricted to the smaller joints such as the wrists, elbows and knees etc. People with this condition often become unable to carry out normal day-to-day activities.

Aromatherapy is very effective in both the treatment and prevention of arthritis.

Oils for Arthritis		
Top	**Middle**	**Base**
Basil*	Black Pepper*	Benzoin
Cajuput	Chamomile*	Cedarwood
Clary Sage*	Clary Sage*	Ginger*
Eucalyptus*	Cypress	Myrrh
Peppermint*	Juniper*	Vetiver
Lemon*	Lavender*	
Thyme*	Marjoram	
	Peppermint*	
	Pine (Scotch)	
	Rosemary*	
	Sweet Fennel*	

Asthma

Asthma affects the passages which take air to the lungs, making them irritated. Asthma can cause wheezing, shortness of breath, coughing, chest tightness and difficulty in speaking.

Often people have problems with breathing out rather than breathing in. Asthma can be bought on by infection or allergy / trigger such as smoke or Hay fever.

Asthma can be life threatening if not treated effectively, and people can become very anxious or frightened during an attack.

It can affect people of any age including young children, and is treated medically with inhalers or oral medicine.

Attacks can also sometimes be controlled with breathing exercises.

Aromatherapy should be used to treat infection where present or to relax the person. If a person is having an asthma attack they should immediately take any medication and use the breathing exercises they have been taught. Aromatherapy cannot be used in place of these at any time.

Oils for Asthma		
Top	**Middle**	**Base**
Basil*	Clary Sage*	Benzoin
Cajuput	Cypress	Frankincense
Clary Sage*	Lavender*	Jasmine*
Eucalyptus*	Marjoram	Myrrh
Lemon*	Melissa	Rose*
Niaouli	Peppermint*	Sandalwood
Peppermint*	Pine (Scotch)	
Tea Tree*	Rosemary*	
Thyme*	Sweet Fennel*	

Athletes Foot

Athletes foot is a fungal infection usually confined to the feet between the toes, caused by a mould or yeast which initially grows on the surface of the skin but then infects the underlying living skin.

The use of essential oils which are fungicidal can be beneficial.

Oils for Athletes Foot		
Top	**Middle**	**Base**
Eucalyptus* Lemon* Lemongrass	Cypress Lavender*	Myrrh Patchouli

Top Tip: The best way to administer the oils for Athletes foot is through a foot bath with warm water in which the oils have been added and dissipated. You can also make a lotion using 5ml of isopropyl alcohol or vodka and adding 6 drops of the essential oil to it.

Bleeding Gums

Also known as gingivitis, this is inflammation of the gums surrounding the teeth, which leads to bleeding.

Usually the person has other illnesses or is taking medication which makes them more susceptible to this condition.

Occasionally pregnancy can cause this condition due to the changes the body is undergoing.

Symptoms include redness, swelling, bleeding and pain in the gums along with bad breath.

People with gingivitis need to see their dentist regularly and use thorough mouth hygiene including mouthwashes and floss.

Oils for Bleeding Gums		
Top	**Middle**	**Base**
Grapefruit	Cypress	Myrrh
Mandarin	Sweet Fennel*	
Tea Tree*		
Thyme*		

Top Tip: Do not brush your teeth hard as this encourages the gums to recede and may give rise to places where infection can breed. If the gums are too sore to brush place a few drops of the mouthwash on your immaculately clean fingertips and gently massage into the gums.

Blocked Nose

A blocked nose is often symptomatic of catarrh build-up.

It is not a condition in its own right but a symptom of something else such as a cold, Hay fever or an allergy.

In some cases a blocked nose can be caused by nasal polyps which need to be diagnosed by a medical practitioner.

If the nose is blocked for any length of time once other symptoms have disappeared, then medical advice should be sought.

Oils for Blocked Noses		
Top	**Middle**	**Base**
Basil*	Lavender*	
Eucalyptus*	Peppermint*	
Grapefruit		
Lemon*		
Lime		
Peppermint*		

Top Tip: You can use Eucalyptus around the nostrils and sinus areas for more severe congestion, but dilute it first in a little carrier oil.

Blood Pressure - High (Hypertension)

High blood pressure is very common although most people will not know that they have it. It occurs when the blood flowing through the arteries meets some resistance. This could be plaque build-up on the inside of the blood vessel or a natural narrowing of the area.

Blood pressure measures the strength of the blood being pumped around the body against the walls of the arteries. If it is too high it puts a strain on the arteries and heart which can lead to other illnesses.

Most people get no symptoms with high blood pressure, but long term complications such as heart attacks or strokes can occur so it is important to treat early.

Contributing factors to high blood pressure can include being overweight, having a family history of hypertension, having a poor diet that lacks vegetables and fruit or is high is salt content, lack of exercise, a high intake of coffee and alcohol, or being over 65 years old.

But it is significant to note that not everyone with hypertension has all or any of these problems.

Medical treatment focuses on reducing any of the above issues that may be present, and prescribing medication where necessary. Aromatherapy oils can also help to lower the pressure due to their chemical components, or to treat the symptoms of breathlessness and anxiety. They are best used as a massage oil.

Oils for High Blood Pressure		
Top	**Middle**	**Base**
Bergamot*	Chamomile*	Frankincense
Clary Sage*	Clary Sage*	Neroli*
Lemon*	Juniper*	Rose*
MayChang (Litsea Cubeba)	Lavender*	Valerian*
	Marjoram	Ylang Ylang
	Melissa	
	Sweet Fennel	

Top Tip: Try to have a bath or massage to get the oils into the bloodstream, and eat a healthier diet which is low in cholesterol.

Blood Pressure - Low (Hypotension)

Low blood pressure is also known as hypotension, which is defined as having a blood pressure reading of below 90/60.

Normally this is not a problem and is actually a sign of good health, but if it drops too low it can restrict the amount of blood going to your brain and other organs. This can cause fainting, dizziness and loss of balance.

When not symptomatic of an underlying condition, low blood pressure is generally considered to be a sign of good health because there is less stress on the heart and blood vessels. Therefore unless you experience lots of dizziness, fainting and unsteadiness there is no need to see your medical practitioner.

Self-help options for low blood pressure include making sure you stand up slowly from sitting; avoiding standing for long periods of time; ensuring you drink plenty of fluids to keep hydrated; adding more salt to your meals and having smaller meals more often; and wearing support stockings to encourage circulation.

Oils for Low Blood Pressure		
Top	**Middle**	**Base**
Peppermint* Thyme*	Black Pepper* Peppermint* Rosemary*	Cinnamon

Top Tip: Rosemary has been used for eons to raise blood pressure to a more normal level, whereas Black Pepper and Peppermint are extremely useful if a person has been fainting a lot. Use a brisker type of massage to administer the oils used as it encourages the circulation of blood around the body.

Catarrh

Catarrh is often linked to the common cold and is characterised by a runny or blocked nose. It can also be associated with Hay fever, sinusitis, tonsillitis or adenoid and ear infections. Sometimes the blockages caused by catarrh can last a long time and become chronic.

Oils for Catarrh		
Top	**Middle**	**Base**
Basil*	Black Pepper*	Benzoin
Bergamot*	Chamomile*	Cedarwood
Eucalyptus*	Juniper*	Frankincense
Lemon*	Lavender*	Ginger*
Niaouli	Marjoram	Jasmine*
Peppermint*	Melissa	Myrrh
Tea Tree*	Peppermint*	Sandalwood
Thyme*	Pine (Scotch)	
	Rosemary*	

Top Tip: Steam inhalations can help really well to ease blockages and fight infection. Massaging the face and down the neck will help drain away the fluids.

Cold Sores / Herpes

Lots of people get cold sores, which are caused by the herpes virus. The first sign of having a cold sore is small blisters that develop on or around the lips and mouth.

These usually clear up of their own accord in seven to ten days.

The problem with the herpes virus is that you may not even know you have caught it. You may have it for a long time before you have your first outbreak. Then you may have one outbreak and never have another one, or have repeated outbreaks; it just depends on the person.

Cold sores start with a tingling, burning or itching sensation in the area affected and then small fluid-filled blisters emerge. Once you have had a first outbreak you usually pick up on the symptoms that indicate another outbreak is coming on, and can start treatment immediately.

Cold sores are highly contagious, so be careful not to kiss or have skin-to-skin contact where the blisters are located.

Start the aromatherapy treatment as soon as the first sign appears.

Oils for Cold Sores		
Top	**Middle**	**Base**
Bergamot*	Lavender*	
Tea Tree*		

Colds

The common cold is the most frequently occurring illness in the whole world, as there are more than 200 different viruses that can cause it.

Cold symptoms will usually last for five to ten days and are mild, but in a few cases the cold can turn into a more serious illness.

The new illness is not the cold virus but another bacterial or viral infection that is caught during this time when the body is already fighting one illness. If this happens then medical attention should be sought and the new illness can then be treated.

Aromatherapy can work very well to help relieve cold symptoms. A number of essential oils can help in different ways to relieve the symptoms of colds, coughs and blocked nose. To help with making a mix for a cold you can refer to the other symptom pages in this book to help choose the exact oils that can help.

The two most useful methods for using essential oils for colds are steam inhalations and baths, although massaging the chest and throat areas can also be beneficial.

Oils for Colds		
Top	**Middle**	**Base**
Basil*	Black Pepper*	Benzoin
Bergamot*	Geranium*	Cedarwood
Cajuput	Juniper*	Cinnamon
Eucalyptus*	Lavender*	Frankincense
Grapefruit	Marjoram	Ginger*
Lemon*	Melissa	Myrrh
Niaouli	Peppermint	
Peppermint*	Pine (Scotch)	
Tea Tree*	Rosemary*	
Thyme*		

Constipation

When people become constipated it is usually because they have not drunk enough water in some form which makes the stools hard and painful. You also do not go to the toilet as much as you usually do.

However, constipation can also be a result of stress, anxiety or other emotional issues. So it is important to get a complete picture of what the person is experiencing right now in their life and treat all the issues -- not just this one.

It is more common in older people, but in some instances constipation is caused by other problems in the bowel. If you are experiencing persistent constipation then see your medical practitioner as soon as possible.

Drink more water and exercise as much as possible in addition to treating them with oils. Massage is the best method of getting the essential oils into the body to treat constipation.

Oils for Constipation		
Top	**Middle**	**Base**
Grapefruit	Black Pepper*	Cinnamon
Lemon*	Chamomile*	Ginger*
Mandarin	Marjoram	Patchouli
	Rosemary*	Rose*
	Sweet Fennel*	

Top Tip: As constipation can sometimes be as a result of stress, anxiety, shock or emotional problems, relaxing treatments using aromatherapy essential oils can be beneficial.

Massage the abdomen in a clockwise direction using essential oils. Some of the best are Black Pepper, Sweet Fennel*, Juniper, Marjoram, Patchouli and Rosemary

Coughs - General

People cough to get rid of mucus or any irritant that they have inhaled such as smoke or dust.

But if you have a persistent cough then it is a symptom of something else. This could be a cold, the flu or another viral or bacterial infection.

Anyone who is coughing for longer than 10 days should see a medical practitioner. This is especially important if they have other issues with their lungs such as asthma or emphysema. If a child has a persistent cough then medical treatment should be sought as it may be symptomatic of whooping cough.

The problem with coughs is that over time the chest becomes sore as the muscles are having to work hard. They can make it hard to breathe especially if asthma or other issues are present.

However, aromatherapy treatments can be very beneficial for coughs as they can sooth the throat, help fight infection, expel mucus, relieve bronchial spasm and induce relaxation.

There are a variety of ways to treat the cough which include massaging the chest, throat and upper back using a blend of essential oils in carrier oil, and steam inhalation which is an excellent way of soothing the throat and bronchi whilst helping to expel mucus.

Oils for Coughs		
Top	**Middle**	**Base**
Clary Sage*	Black Pepper*	Benzoin
Eucalyptus*	Carrot Seed	Cedarwood
Lemon*	Clary Sage*	Cinnamon
Niaouli	Cypress	Frankincense
Peppermint*	Juniper*	Ginger*
Thyme*	Lavender*	Jasmine*
	Melissa	Myrrh
	Peppermint*	Rose*
	Pine (Scotch)	Sandalwood
	Rosemary*	

Top Tip: Essential oils such as Benzoin, Chamomile (Roman), Eucalyptus, Frankincense, Lavender, Marjoram, Rosemary, Sandalwood, Tea Tree and Thyme are all really good for coughs. When the chest feels tight and it is hard to cough then steam inhalations can relieve this feeling.

Cracked Dry Skin

Anyone who has had cracked dry skin or lips will know how painful it can be and how sensitive the area gets. Lips can continually crack whilst talking, eating or drinking.

However the dryness is often caused by evaporation of moisture from the skin because of exposure to heat or cold, or because of the wind. It is important to drink as much as possible if you have dry cracked skin or lips to replace the moisture lost from your skin. In addition, you can try any of the following oils to help nourish the area.

Oils for Cracked Dry Skin		
Top	**Middle**	**Base**
	Carrot Seed	Benzoin
	Chamomile (Roman)*	Jasmine*
	Geranium*	Myrrh
	Lavender*	Neroli*
	Marjoram	Patchouli
	Sweet Fennel*	Rose*
		Sandalwood

Top Tip: Regular massage into the chapped skin will help the circulation in the tiny blood vessels and will help to nourish and lubricate. The best way to get the oils into your skin or lips is to mix them into cream (hand or body) and applying them straight onto the area.

Cramp

When muscles shorten or contract sometimes they cause pain which is unpleasant or severe in the area affected. This is known as cramp. Cramps can occur in the extremities such as legs, or in other areas of the body such as the stomach or lower abdomen. Causes of cramp include dehydration, low salt or oxygen levels in the blood, over-extension of a muscle, or sudden changes in temperature. Sometimes cramps can be symptomatic of other diseases.

The most common types of cramp include:

<u>Menstrual cramps</u> for women, which can vary in severity. These cramps tend to be in the lower abdomen and radiate through to the lower back and thighs. Most often tablets such as ibuprofen and paracetamol can help along with warm baths and heat to the area. See the entry for dysmenorrhea for more information.

<u>Skeletal cramps</u> which occur most often in the muscles of the calves, thighs, feet.

Oils for Cramp		
Top	**Middle**	**Base**
Clary Sage*	Chamomile (Roman)*	Ginger*
Peppermint*	Clary Sage*	
	Cypress	
	Frankincense	
	Geranium*	
	Lavender*	
	Marjoram	
	Peppermint*	
	Rosemary*	

Top Tip: If you have regular cramps try bathing your legs and feet in a bath with oils for at least 30 minutes.

Cuts

A cut is an opening in the skin typically caused by a sharp object which has penetrated through and separated the outer layers of skin, causing bleeding. The skin has not been removed such as happens with a graze or friction-type injury. In medical terms there are several ways to describe the cut and what it looks like: A jagged-edged cut tends to be called a laceration and a deeper and longer cut is known as a gash.

If pressure is applied to a cut it usually stops bleeding within a few minutes. If it continues, or the blood spurts out, then medical attention is needed immediately.

There are several essential oils that can help with minor cuts, but it is important to ensure the area is clean and free from dirt as much as possible before putting them on.

Oils for Cuts		
Top	**Middle**	**Base**
Eucalyptus*	Chamomile*	Vetiver
Lemon*	Lavender*	
Niaouli	Pine (Scotch)	
Tea Tree*		

Top Tip: If you intend to put a plaster onto a cut, put one drop of lavender essential oil onto the plaster before application

Cystitis

Cystitis is inflammation of the bladder and can be caused by bacteria, injury or trauma.

Symptoms include a frequent need to wee and / or pain on passing urine.

It is important to treat cystitis, as prolonged periods can lead to the infection travelling up to the kidneys, producing a more painful and serious condition.

Cystitis is more common in women, and children or men with the condition should always be referred to a medical practitioner.

Mild cystitis usually clears up in four to nine days and people are encouraged to drink six to eight glasses of water a day to help clear the infection and take normal painkillers.

Oils for Cystitis		
Top	**Middle**	**Base**
Bergamot*	Black Pepper*	Benzoin
Cajuput	Carrot Seed	Cedarwood
Eucalyptus*	Chamomile (Roman)*	Frankincense
Niaouli	Juniper*	Sandalwood
Tea Tree*	Lavender*	
Thyme*	Parsley	
	Pine (Scotch)	
	Sweet Fennel*	

Depression

Depression is the term given to feelings of extreme sadness that can last for a long time to the extent that these feelings can disrupt daily living. In extreme cases people feel unable to live any longer, have thoughts of suicide and need professional help quickly.

It is totally different from the common feelings of being miserable or feeling unhappy over a short period of time. It is estimated that one in ten people will experience depression at some point in their life, including in childhood.

Aromatherapy treatment tends to assist with the symptoms that accompany depression such as insomnia, so a full discussion of what other symptoms the person is experiencing will enable treatment to be tailored to their individual need.

Oils for Depression		
Top	**Middle**	**Base**
Basil*	Chamomile*	Cinnamon
Bergamot*	Clary Sage*	Frankincense
Clary Sage*	Geranium*	Ginger*
Eucalyptus*	Lavender*	Jasmine*
Grapefruit	Melissa	Neroli*
Lemon*		Patchouli
Petitgrain		Rose
Thyme*		Sandalwood
		Vetiver
		Ylang Ylang

Dermatitis / Eczema

Dermatitis is also known as eczema, a condition which can cause the skin in any area to become itchy, flaky, dry and red, sometimes making cracks appear. It can be sore and irritating, and quite upsetting if it is in places other people can see.

There are several different forms:

<u>Atopic eczema</u> is mostly found in children, who often grow out of the condition. It is commonly found behind the knees, elbows, neck and face, and can be light or severe. It is thought to affect children who also experience asthma and Hay fever, or who have other members of the family with the same condition.

<u>Contact dermatitis</u> is caused through contact with an irritant or a substance the person is allergic to. Anyone can experience contact dermatitis.

<u>Discord eczema</u> is a long-lasting condition with oval or circular shaped patches of eczema of any size. It must be treated by a medical practitioner as it can take years to clear, often re-occurring. It is more common in men over 50 and young women.

<u>Varicose eczema</u> affects the skin around and over varicose veins. Treatment of this condition usually involves treating the varicose veins at the same time.

<u>Seborrheic dermatitis</u> is the commonest cause of and makes the skin inflamed or itchy. However, in addition

to the scalp this condition can also be found on the face, ears, chest, shoulder blades, and creases of the skin such as behind the knees. Commonly the skin flakes, weeps and forms scales that are either yellow or white.

Oils for Dermatitis / Eczema		
Top	**Middle**	**Base**
Bergamot*	Chamomile*	Benzoin
Clary Sage*	Cypress	Cedarwood
MayChang (Litsea Cubeba)	Geranium*	Jasmine*
	Juniper*	Myrrh
Peppermint*	Lavender*	Patchouli
Thyme*	Melissa	Rose*
	Peppermint*	Sandalwood
	Pine (Scotch)	
	Rosemary*	

Diarrhoea

Diarrhoea is something most people experience at some time in their lives. Medically speaking it is the passing of loose, often watery, stools more than three times a day.

It is only concerning if it continues for a few weeks, or more than five days in very young children and babies.

Although commonly caused by a viral or bacterial infection, it can also be experienced by people under stress or who are very anxious.

It can also be a side effect of some medication such as antibiotics.

People with diarrhoea should ensure that they drink plenty of fluids containing sugar (but no caffeine as that can cause dehydration), and avoid products containing lactose whilst ill. Normal food, excluding lactose, can be taken during this time.

Oils for Diarrhoea		
Top	**Middle**	**Base**
Eucalyptus*	Benzoin	Cinnamon
Lemon*	Black Pepper*	Ginger*
Mandarin	Carrot Seed	Myrrh
Niaouli	Chamomile*	Neroli*
Peppermint*	Cypress	Patchouli
Tea Tree*	Geranium*	Sandalwood
	Juniper*	
	Lavender*	
	Peppermint*	
	Rosemary*	

Earache

Earache is very common in children and can be very painful. Causes include an infection in the middle or outer ear, a condition called 'glue ear', eczema, a scrap in the ear, earwax or as a side effect of another infection such as tonsillitis.

Most ear infections clear up on their own but medical treatment should be sought. Aromatherapy treatment can be carried out alongside any medical treatment prescribed.

Oils for Earache		
Top	**Middle**	**Base**
Basil*	Chamomile*	Rose*
Cajuput	Lavender*	
Niaouli	Peppermint*	
Peppermint*	Rosemary*	

Flatulence

Flatulence is the wind or gas that is passed through the gut and out of the rectum. It is frequently called 'trumping' or 'farting' and is the subject of many a school yard joke all over the world.

But everyone does it on average 15 times a day. (Even the Queen!)

Often the gas is odourless but sometimes there is a smell accompanying it.

This is due to undigested food that is beginning to decompose in the intestines.

Causes of flatulence include swallowing more air than usual when eating or eating food that is hard to digest or that the body is not used to.

Whilst not harmful, flatulence can be socially embarrassing.

Therefore some methods of reducing flatulence can be made through changing dietary habits by eating more natural yoghurt and drinking plenty of water.

Oils for Flatulence		
Top	**Middle**	**Base**
Basil*	Black Pepper*	Benzoin
Bergamot*	Carrot Seed	Cinnamon

<table>
<tr><th colspan="3" align="center">Oils for Flatulence</th></tr>
<tr><th align="center">Top</th><th align="center">Middle</th><th align="center">Base</th></tr>
<tr><td align="center">Clary Sage*</td><td align="center">Chamomile*</td><td align="center">Ginger*</td></tr>
<tr><td align="center">Lemon*</td><td align="center">Clary Sage*</td><td align="center">Myrrh</td></tr>
<tr><td align="center">Mandarin</td><td align="center">Geranium*</td><td align="center">Neroli*</td></tr>
<tr><td align="center">MayChang (Litsea Cubeba)</td><td align="center">Juniper*</td><td align="center"></td></tr>
<tr><td align="center"></td><td align="center">Lavender*</td><td align="center"></td></tr>
<tr><td align="center">Peppermint*</td><td align="center">Marjoram</td><td align="center"></td></tr>
<tr><td align="center">Petitgrain</td><td align="center">Melissa</td><td align="center"></td></tr>
<tr><td align="center">Thyme*</td><td align="center">Peppermint*</td><td align="center"></td></tr>
<tr><td align="center"></td><td align="center">Sweet Fennel*</td><td align="center"></td></tr>
</table>

Top Tip: Essential oils described as 'carminative' will help to expel gas from the digestive system and ease the pain which accompanies it.

Massage the essential oils diluted in carrier oil into the abdomen working round the tummy in a clockwise direction.

Flu

Flu is a highly contagious viral illness often confused with the common cold, as symptoms tend to be more severe and last longer (up to 10 days or more).

There are more than 200 viruses that cause flu, but not all are around at the same time. In fact flu can be caught all year round, but is especially common in winter.

Symptoms of the flu include high temperatures, headaches, joint aches and pains, sore throat and weakness. This can also be accompanied by a cough.

The best treatment in most cases is to remain in bed avoiding physical exercise, smoking and alcohol, and take medicines that reduce temperatures.

There are some aromatherapy treatments that can also help, but medical treatment should be sought if there are complications such as a chest infection, you have an underlying medical condition, are over 65, or are pregnant.

There are no cures for flu, although in some instances antiviral medicine can be prescribed. Those in high risk groups in the UK are offered seasonal vaccinations in the autumn, which can prevent some instances of flu which have been predicted to be prevalent that season.

Oils for Flu		
Top	**Middle**	**Base**
Basil*	Black Pepper*	Benzoin
Bergamot*	Chamomile*	Cedarwood
Eucalyptus*	Cypress	Cinnamon

Oils for Flu		
Top	**Middle**	**Base**
Grapefruit	Geranium*	Ginger*
Lemon*	Juniper*	Frankincense
Niaouli	Lavender*	Sandalwood
Peppermint*	Peppermint*	
Tea Tree*	Pine (Scotch)	
Thyme*	Rosemary*	

Top Tip: Have a hotish bath and add oils to make a steam inhalation. Alternatively use oils in an oil burner in the sick person's room. Treat the symptoms as well as the actual flu itself.

Fluid Retention / Oedema

Lots of people get fluid retention at some time in their life. Known as oedema, the swelling can take place in a localised area such as the ankles, or it can affect larger parts of the body and in some cases the whole body.

Women often get fluid retention before their menstrual cycle starts. This can be helped with massage in the seven to ten days before the menstruation starts.

Aeroplanes and flying can be blamed for some oedema, where the legs and ankles swell. Some people have to wear special flight socks to stop it happening, but sometimes massaging the area with essential oils before and during the flight can help too.

Even people who have to stand for long periods of time can have episodes of fluid retention and can benefit from aromatherapy treatment.

Oils for Oedema		
Top	**Middle**	**Base**
Bergamot*	Black Pepper*	Benzoin
Clary Sage*	Carrot Seed	Cedarwood
Eucalyptus*	Chamomile*	Frankincense
Grapefruit	Clary Sage*	Patchouli
Lemon*	Cypress	Sandalwood
Mandarin	Geranium*	Valerian*
Petitgrain	Juniper*	
Thyme*	Lavender*	
	Rosemary*	
	Sweet Fennel*	

Top Tip: Massage the legs from the ankles upwards to encourage the fluid to drain away.

Gastroenteritis

Otherwise known as diarrhoea and vomiting, gastroenteritis is a very common condition usually caused by bacteria or a virus.

When children get gastroenteritis it is most commonly the rotavirus that they contract, but adults tend to have the notorious norovirus.

Other causes include food poisoning.

Having diarrhoea and vomiting is quite unpleasant, but it usually clears up within a week, and most people can stay at home until it has cleared up. It is important not to mix with other people for at least 48 hours after the last bout of diarrhoea and/or vomiting, which is why children are not allowed to go back to school until this time has passed, as it can be very contagious.

The typical symptoms of gastroenteritis are sudden watery poos with stomach cramps, feeling sick, vomiting (sometimes projectile), and a mild temperature. You might also get a headache and feel very off your food.

It is important to drink plenty of water to keep yourself hydrated during this time, as dehydration is the most common reason for hospitalisation.

Oils for Gastroenteritis		
Top	**Middle**	**Base**
Basil*	Chamomile*	Sandalwood
Bergamot*	Geranium*	Ylang Ylang
Cajuput	Lavender*	
Lemongrass	Peppermint*	
Niaouli	Pine (Scotch)	
Peppermint*	Rosemary*	
Tea Tree*		
Thyme*		

Top Tip: Burning oils in an oil burner in the person's room can help, as can gentle massage with oils on the tummy area.

Gout

Gout is a common type of arthritis where the body has built up too much uric acid and cannot remove it. Uric acid is the waste product produced when the body breaks down food for energy. It is excreted through the kidneys, and if the body is not getting rid of the acid or over-producing it, the levels become very high and form crystals in the joints, causing swelling and intense pain.

It mainly affects men aged between 40 – 60 and women after their menopause (60-80).

Unfortunately any joint can be affected, but it usually affects areas such as the toes, ankles, knees and fingers. The joints become hot, swollen and painful with tight, shiny skin over the top. This develops rapidly and usually lasts for up to 10 days.

The first attack of gout will stop after two to three weeks, but subsequent attacks can become more frequent over time and last longer and longer, and affect more than one or two joints.

Alcohol, red meat and seafood can make the condition worse, so a change in diet can help. Many people find that they can rid themselves of the disease completely over time by making changes to their diet and cutting down on alcohol.

Oils for Gout		
Top	**Middle**	**Base**
Basil*	Black Pepper*	Benzoin
Cajuput	Chamomile*	Frankincense
Eucalyptus*	Geranium*	Ginger*
Lemon*	Juniper*	Sandalwood
Mandarin	Lavender*	
Peppermint*	Marjoram	
Thyme*	Peppermint*	
	Pine (Scotch)	
	Rosemary*	

Haemorrhoids

Anyone with haemorrhoids knows that this is a condition that can be very painful, yet people seldom talk about it. This is because haemorrhoids are enlarged veins in your bottom, either inside or outside. Sometimes if they are outside they can resemble grapes and bleed when you got to the toilet or wipe your bottom.

Treatment varies dependant on the severity of the haemorrhoids, from creams to surgery, so it is important to get a medical opinion as well as treating with aromatherapy oils.

There are steps that can be taken to relieve the symptoms along with the aromatherapy techniques and oils.

The best self-help treatment is to drink more liquids, and eat more green vegetables, as constipation is the most likely cause of haemorrhoids. Try not to strain when you open your bowels.

Stool softeners, or over-the-counter creams specifically made for haemorrhoids may assist in reducing pain and swelling, and sitting on a round cushion with a hole in the centre like a swimming ring may be more comfortable.

Oils for Haemorrhoids		
Top	**Middle**	**Base**
	Cypress	Frankincense
	Geranium*	Myrrh
	Juniper*	
	Marjoram	
	Rosemary*	
	Sweet Fennel	

Top Tip: Try using a Sitz baths for 15 minutes three times a day and after each bowel movement, ensuring that the skin around the anus is thoroughly dried by patting dry. Massaging with Fennel, Marjoram and Rosemary over the abdomen in a clockwise direction can also help.

Headaches

Everyone gets a headache now and then and the causes can be very general, from straining the eyes when reading to not drinking enough fluid. These are not migraines but general headaches that focus in the head. They may also spread out to the muscles around the head, neck, and shoulders.

The head pain may be in the temples, forehead or on both sides of the head and may be mild or moderate.

Severe pain resulting in nausea, vomiting or sensitivity to sound or light is more likely to be classed as migraine.

If the pain spreads out to the shoulders then you have a tension headache which is usually the result of stress. If a headache is present for more than 15 days per month or longer than six months, you have a chronic headache and you should see a medical practitioner.

Alternatively tension headaches could be the result of sinusitis or catarrh.

Oils for Headaches		
Top	**Middle**	**Base**
Basil*	Black Pepper*	Rose*
Cajuput	Chamomile*	
Eucalyptus*	Marjoram	
Grapefruit	Melissa	
Lemongrass	Peppermint*	
Peppermint*	Rosemary*	

Heartburn

Heartburn is a feeling of burning in the chest and stomach area, and is common amongst the adult population. It can feel as though you have something stuck half way down your throat.

It is caused by excess stomach acid and can be associated with certain foods or stress.

Continual bouts can be symptoms of another condition called gastroesophageal reflux and should be treated by a qualified medical practitioner.

It is often said that sipping an infusion made of fennel or peppermint can help with heartburn and indigestion.

Note: Sometimes the pain of heartburn can be confused with more serious heart problems. If the pain is accompanied by sweating, feeling sick, vomiting or breathing problems then call the ambulance immediately.

Oils for Heartburn		
Top	**Middle**	**Base**
Basil*	Black Pepper*	Ginger*
Bergamot*	Carrot Seed	Rose*
Lemon*	Chamomile*	Sandalwood
Peppermint*	Juniper*	
	Lavender*	
	Marjoram	
	Melissa	
	Rosemary*	
	Spearmint	
	Sweet Fennel	

Top Tip: Gently massaging over the stomach area can help; or make a hot compress and place over the stomach area.

High Temperature

A high temperature can also be called a fever, and is caused by your body fighting an infection somewhere.

Your normal temperature is around 36°C – 37°C and anything above 37.5°C is classed as having a high temperature.

If you have a high temperature it usually lasts around two to three days. Make sure you drink plenty of water, wear loose cotton clothes where possible, use sheets rather than duvets or blankets and open the windows to let fresh air in.

The first sign of a temperature can be feeling cold and shivery. Don't give in to it by lying under loads of duvets!

Fevers in children are very common. They are also the most common reason for children visiting their doctor.

If your child has a high temperature then there are three things you can do to help:

Reduce the temperature to under 38°C.

Make sure they are rehydrated.

Monitor them for more serious illnesses.

If the temperature does not start to decrease or reaches a critical level then seek medical attention.

Aromatherapy can help to start the process of reducing your temperature. The best method of using them is in a cold compress.

Oils for a High Temperature		
Top	**Middle**	**Base**
Bergamot*	Chamomile*	
Eucalyptus*	Lavender*	
Lemon*	Melissa	
Lemongrass	Peppermint*	
Niaouli		
Peppermint*		
Tea Tree*		

Indigestion / Dyspepsia

Indigestion is also known as dyspepsia, a term given to pain or discomfort in the stomach area, sometimes combined with feeling bloated, heartburn, burping, swelling of the abdomen, and occasionally feeling sick.

It is a very common condition, causing discomfort in the stomach area or under the diaphragm. Often caused by certain food, stress, tension or anxiety, it is important to get the person afflicted to relax through baths or massage.

If the person is experiencing prolonged episodes, very regular and/or painful episodes, or have it for the first time, they should see their medical practitioner.

Aromatherapy treatments can work for indigestion in two ways. The first is that massage and the use of essential oils can help relax anyone who is tense, anxious or stressed. Massage gently over the stomach, ribcage and throat area.

Alternatively make a hot compress and place over the stomach.

Oils for Indigestion		
Top	**Middle**	**Base**
Basil*	Black Pepper*	Cinnamon
Bergamot*	Carrot Seed	Frankincense
Cajuput	Chamomile*	Ginger*
Clary Sage*	Clary Sage*	Myrrh
Eucalyptus*	Juniper*	Neroli*
Lemon*	Lavender*	Rose
Lemongrass	Marjoram	
Mandarin	Melissa	
MayChang (Litsea Cubeba)	Peppermint*	
	Rosemary*	
Niaouli	Spearmint	
Petitgrain	Sweet Fennel	

Top Tip: Sometimes drinking Chamomile, Fennel* and Peppermint herbal infusions can bring relief.

Insect Stings / Bites

Most bites and stings are methods of defence from the creature involved.

Most people during their lifetime would experience an insect bite or sting. They usually result in swelling and redness.

Some people are allergic to certain stings and can have life-threatening reactions which must be treated medically as quickly as possible.

On bites which are more minor, essential oils can bring some relief from the itching, pain and swelling.

Oils for Insect Stings / Bites		
Top	**Middle**	**Base**
Basil*	Chamomile*	Benzoin
Bergamot*	Clary Sage*	Myrrh
Cajuput	Geranium*	Neroli*
Clary Sage*	Lavender*	Patchouli
Eucalyptus*	Melissa	Rose*
Lemon*	Peppermint*	Ylang Ylang
Niaouli	Spearmint	
Peppermint*	Sweet Fennel	
Tea Tree*		
Thyme*		

<table><tr><td>

Top Tip: Spearmint applied neat onto a sting or bite will instantly stop the itching. However, do not allow this oil to go near the genital area, so wash hands thoroughly after use and do not apply to any of these areas.

</td></tr></table>

Irritable Bowel Syndrome (IBS)

Irritable bowel syndrome affects about one in five people at some time in their life, often developing when they are in their 20s or 30s, with more women than men getting it.

Bouts of IBS tend to come and go, with periods lasting from a few days to a few months.

Symptoms include stomach cramps and lower abdomen cramps or pain, bloating of the stomach and gas (flatulence), along with alternating periods of diarrhoea and constipation.

Symptoms can vary from person to person.

The actual cause of IBS is currently unknown, but it is more common at times of stress or after eating certain foods.

Aromatherapy can help to relieve tension and provide relaxation to the muscles as well as the whole person. Gentle massage around the abdomen and bathing in oils can provide relief from the pain.

Oils for IBS		
Top	**Middle**	**Base**
Eucalyptus*	Black Pepper*	Benzoin
Peppermint*	Chamomile*	Ginger*
	Lavender*	Neroli*
	Peppermint*	
	Sweet Fennel	

Laryngitis

Laryngitis is inflammation of the vocal cords, or larynx.

When someone has laryngitis they may experience loss of voice, hoarseness, mild temperature, an irritating cough and sore throats.

The symptoms usually start quickly and get worse over two or three days, but in most cases it will get better without treatment in about a week. However the hoarseness and loss of voice can continue for a while afterwards.

Laryngitis can be accompanied with other illnesses such as tonsillitis, throat infections or even the flu, so other symptoms may also be present.

Aromatherapy can help with this condition and also any other infections that might be present.

Oils for Laryngitis		
Top	**Middle**	**Base**
Cajuput	Cypress	Benzoin
Eucalyptus*	Lavender*	Frankincense
Thyme*		Jasmine*
		Sandalwood

Migraine

Migraine headaches usually come on as severe pain in the head, often over one or both eyes and the forehead. They can be accompanied by photosensitivity (light sensitivity) and nausea / vomiting.

Classic migraines can have pre-headache symptoms which can warn the person of the oncoming migraine.

These can include partial or full loss of vision, 'flickering' lights (often described as 'bunting' or triangles) in the visual field and, in some cases, strange smells.

Each symptom is individual to the person.

Migraines can vary in frequency from daily to less than one per year, and typically last between four and 72 hours.

Aromatherapy is often better as a preventative measure and is best used as soon as the sufferer feels that the attack is about to commence.

Oils for Migraines		
Top	**Middle**	**Base**
Basil*	Chamomile*	
Clary Sage*	Clary Sage*	
Peppermint*	Lavender*	
	Marjoram	
	Melissa	
	Peppermint*	

Top Tip: Lying in a dark room can help, as can cold compresses, with the oils, placed over the forehead and temples (changing them as soon as they get warm). Some people find relief from using warm compresses across the back of the neck. If the migraine is due to stress, massaging across the neck and shoulders can help to relieve tension.

Mouth Ulcers

Mouth ulcers are painful sores inside the mouth on the cheeks or gums.

They can be caused by biting yourself on the inside of the mouth or as a side effect of medication.

They usually appear red or yellow in colour and can cause a lot of pain and last for between a week and 10 days.

Gentle massage of the gums with a mouthwash will improve local circulation and help to speed up healing.

Oils for Mouth Ulcers		
Top	**Middle**	**Base**
Grapefruit	Peppermint*	Benzoin
Lemon*	Sweet Fennel	Myrrh
Mandarin		
Peppermint*		
Thyme*		

Top Tip: If the gums are too sore to brush, make sure your hands are immaculately clean and put a mix of oils on your fingers, massaging this into the gum area. Myrrh is fantastic for healing ulcers. It can be applied to a cotton bud tip and massaged directly onto the mouth ulcer. Do not swallow this or any other mouthwash you use.

Muscular Aches & Pains

The term muscular aches and pains can cover a myriad of conditions anywhere in the body, ranging from overworked muscles to viruses or cancer of the bones. It is also known as myalgia.

The most common reason for having muscle pain is because you have overworked or over-stretched them somehow.

Whilst there are a variety of treatments available for this condition the underlying condition must also be treated if there is one. Get medical advice if the pain continues for a long period of time.

Physiotherapy is often recommended for people with both chronic and acute muscular pains, depending on the cause.

However, nothing beats a good massage with aromatherapy oils for one-off occasions.

Oils for Muscular Aches & Pains		
Top	**Middle**	**Base**
Basil*	Black Pepper*	Ginger*
Bergamot*	Chamomile*	Jasmine*
Cajuput	Clary Sage*	Neroli*
Clary Sage*	Cypress	Sandalwood
Eucalyptus*	Geranium*	Vetiver
Lemongrass	Juniper*	
Niaouli	Lavender*	
Peppermint*	Marjoram	
Thyme*	Melissa	
	Peppermint*	
	Pine (Scotch)	
	Rosemary*	
	Sweet Fennel	

Top Tip: Epsom salts are good for muscular pain. Relax in a hot bath with a cup of Epsom salts, a cup of sea salt and the aromatherapy oils of your choice for around 20 minutes to help ease the muscles.

Nausea

Nausea and vomiting are common conditions that often go along with many illnesses and diseases. Everyone gets an attack of nausea and vomiting at some time in their lives.

It can be connected with viruses such as the norovirus, or bacteria associated with food poisoning. If the symptoms are accompanied by diarrhoea, ensure that everyone around the sick person washes their hands really well and keeps away from other people for 48 hours after the last bout.

Nausea and vomiting can also be caused by seasickness and motion sickness - from imbalances in the inner ear - cancer therapy, and even stress.

If the vomiting is very severe the person can become dehydrated, so it is important to try to drink plenty of fluids.

See also the entry for vomiting.

Oils for Nausea		
Top	**Middle**	**Base**
Basil*	Black Pepper*	Ginger*
Clary Sage*	Chamomile*	Rose*
Grapefruit	Clary Sage*	Sandalwood
Lemon*	Juniper*	
Mandarin	Lavender*	
Peppermint*	Melissa	
	Peppermint*	

Oils for Nausea		
Top	**Middle**	**Base**
	Sweet Fennel	

Top Tip: Massaging the stomach with the essential oils can help, or alternatively use a warm compress over the area.

Palpitations

Most people at some stage in their lives experience palpitations.

It can be described as feeling as though their heart is missing a beat, fluttering, or speeding / racing.

There may be many causes of palpitations including fear and stress.

However, if these episodes continue for long periods or happen often, then medical attention is required.

Massage with calming aromatherapy oils on a regular basis can help, as it can slow the heart beat down and relax the person experiencing them.

Oils for Palpitations		
Top	**Middle**	**Base**
Eucalyptus*	Chamomile*	Neroli*
Mandarin	Lavender*	Rose*
Peppermint*	Melissa	Ylang Ylang
Thyme*	Peppermint*	
	Rosemary*	

Top Tip: Out of this list of essential oils Ylang Ylang is probably the best one to help to slow the rapid beating of the heart.

Premenstrual Tension (PMT) or Premenstrual Syndrome (PMS)

These names are given to the symptoms experienced by women in the days leading up to their periods or menstruation.

Symptoms can include pain, irritability, headaches and migraines, tender breasts, mood swings and hot flushes, but symptoms are unique to the individual. Not everyone has the same ones.

The symptoms usually improve once bleeding has commenced, and disappear after a few days.

PMS/PMT can coincide with menstrual cramps (dysmenorrhea).

Oils for PMS / PMT		
Top	**Middle**	**Base**
Bergamot*	Carrot Seed	Benzoin
Clary Sage*	Chamomile*	Cedarwood
Grapefruit	Clary Sage*	Frankincense
Lemon*	Cypress	Jasmine*
Lemongrass	Geranium*	Neroli*
	Juniper*	Rose*
	Lavender*	Sandalwood
	Marjoram	Ylang Ylang
	Melissa	
	Parsley	
	Rosemary*	
	Sweet Fennel	

Top Tip: Aromatherapy oils can help relieve the symptoms. Ensure you look up all the symptoms related to the person you are treating for this condition and pick oils that will help with them all. Have a warm bath on a regular basis and use a combination of any of the above oils.

Rheumatism

Rheumatism is a generic term used for conditions which cause chronic (long term) or intermittent pain in the joints or connective tissue.

It is an umbrella term for up to 200 different diseases, but they all have two things in common: chronic pain (even if intermittent) and difficulty in treating.

The major types of rheumatism include ankylosing spondylitis, back pain, tendonitis, bursitis, neck pain, osteoarthritis, and rheumatoid arthritis (see separate entry).

Aromatherapy can help with the pain and inflammation associated with these rheumatic disorders. The best methods of using the oils in this situation include compresses and baths.

Oils for Rheumatism		
Top	**Middle**	**Base**
Basil*	Black Pepper*	Benzoin
Cajuput	Chamomile*	Cedarwood
Eucalyptus*	Cypress	Cinnamon
Lemon*	Juniper*	Ginger*
Niaouli	Lavender*	Vetiver
	Marjoram	
	Pine (Scotch)	

Oils for Rheumatism		
Top	**Middle**	**Base**
	Rosemary* Sweet Fennel	

Scars

Scars are part of the body's natural healing process, usually where skin, muscle and soft tissue knit back together after a tear, injury or cut.

They can occur both inside and outside the body.

The type of scar is dependent on the individual as some people are prone to thickening of scars whereas other people heal very well and are left with small, thin scars. Scars usually turn silver over time, but can still burn in the sun.

Stretch marks are also scars but these tend to occur after pregnancy, weight loss, and weight gain or even during growth spurts when children are growing quickly.

Even wrinkles are classed as scars, even though they are mostly part of getting older.

Some people are very anxious or upset about the appearance of scars and it is important to gauge their emotional feelings about the scars and treat the emotion as well.

Bio oil is known to have significant effects on reducing the look and feel of scars, but other aromatherapy oils can also help and assist the skin in healing more effectively.

Oils for Scars		
Top	**Middle**	**Base**
Mandarin	Carrot Seed	Frankincense
Tea Tree*	Chamomile*	Jasmine*
	Geranium*	Myrrh
	Juniper*	Neroli*
	Lavender*	Patchouli
		Rose*
		Sandalwood

Sciatica

Sciatica is the name given to the pain that results from pressure on the sciatic nerve. This nerve runs from the spinal cord through the bottom and down the back of each leg.

Where each nerve leaves the safety of the spinal cord and spinal column there are six or seven nerve roots, and pressure to any of these will result in sciatica.

The severity of the condition can range from mild lower back aches or aches in the buttocks through to severe pain. You may feel pain while moving or walking, numbness down the leg and into the foot, or even loss of muscle power.

Sciatica can last a few hours to a few days depending on the cause, but in more severe cases medical attention should be sought to identify the specific reason for the pressure.

Oils for Sciatica		
Top	**Middle**	**Base**
Eucalyptus* Peppermint*	Chamomile* Lavender* Peppermint*	

Top Tip: When the pain is severe massage is not advisable so use cold compresses over the painful area. Gentle massage is suitable for mild pain. Baths can also help immensely.

Sinusitis

Sinusitis is the inflammation of the sinuses and lining of the nose, which can cause headaches and pressure in the face including eyes, nose, forehead, and cheeks.

Most people get it at some time in their lives.

It can occur on either or both sides of the head and can often be linked to colds, coughs, temperatures, blocked noses and catarrh.

Sinusitis can be acute with sudden onset, or chronic over a long period of time.

Facial massage can sometimes help drain away any fluids trapped in the sinuses, and steam inhalations five to six times a day with the oils can help immensely.

Oils for Sinusitis		
Top	**Middle**	**Base**
Basil*	Lavender*	Ginger*
Eucalyptus*	Peppermint*	
Niaouli	Pine (Scotch)	
Peppermint*		
Tea Tree*		
Thyme*		

Top Tip: Garlic capsules are great for sinusitis. Take regularly as a supplement if possible, or include lots of garlic in your diet.

Sore Throats / Pharyngitis

Pharyngitis is a common condition caused by a variety of viruses and bacteria.

It can also be a symptom of other illnesses such as colds and flu, upper and lower respiratory tract infections, tonsillitis or quinsy, mumps, measles, chickenpox, glandular fever, scarlet fever, rubella (German measles) etc.

Your throat becomes sore to swallow, you may be hoarse and it might hurt to talk.

To soothe the throat, steam inhalations can be used along with a gargle of honey, lemon and sea salt.

Oils for Sore Throats		
Top	**Middle**	**Base**
Niaouli	Lavender*	Benzoin
Thyme*	Pine (Scotch)	Sandalwood

Spasms / Muscle Cramps

Muscle cramps and spasms are caused by the tightening and shortening of muscles, which can last from a few seconds to many minutes.

The body has no control over these spasms and the muscle feels hard and very painful.

Most people will get some form of muscle cramp at some time. It may be caused by over-exercise or a lack of salt, but often it happens for no apparent reason at all.

Muscle cramps are most common in the legs and feet but can occur in any of the extremities, leaving the affected area tender for up to 24 hours afterwards.

Oils for Spasms / Muscle Cramps		
Top	**Middle**	**Base**
Basil*	Black Pepper*	Cinnamon
Bergamot*	Chamomile*	Jasmine*
Cajuput	Clary Sage*	Neroli*
Clary Sage*	Cypress	Rose*
Eucalyptus*	Juniper*	Sandalwood
Peppermint*	Lavender*	Valerian*
Thyme*	Marjoram	
	Peppermint*	
	Rosemary*	
	Sweet Fennel	

Top Tip: Use hot compresses over the affected area, combining this with gentle massage. Remember to warm up muscles before any type of exercise which may help prevent the cramps from occurring.

Stiffness

Stiffness is an overall term for both joint and muscle pain. Assistance for joint stiffness can be found under the entries for rheumatism and rheumatoid arthritis, so this section deals with muscle stiffness.

Muscle stiffness occurs in everyone at some stage or other. It can vary in intensity from just being stiff in the morning to a debilitating pain where you cannot move.

Muscle pain can occur practically anywhere in the body and is often caused by overworking the muscles in exercise, muscle tension, or straining the muscle through work activity.

Not all muscle pain can be attributed to these though, and if you consider that the pain is not down to one of the three above mentioned causes it might be worth seeing if there is another illness to consider. For example, having a temperature can make your muscles feel stiff.

If it's a sprain or a strain then use ice on the affected area for at least three days, and rest. If it's due to over-exertion then avoid the activity that caused it, use gentle stretching exercises and try a low impact type of exercise such as yoga.

Oils for Stiffness		
Top	**Middle**	**Base**
Grapefruit	Black Pepper*	Jasmine*
Thyme*	Cypress	Vetiver
	Lavender*	
	Marjoram	
	Rosemary*	

Stomach Ache

Everyone gets stomach ache at some time. It can be a sharp pain, a dull ache, or cramps, but it usually gets better quickly within a few hours at the most.

If your stomach is bloated you probably have trapped wind. If it is accompanied by diarrhoea then you may have gastroenteritis.

However, if it continues then you should seek medical attention to rule out any major issue.

Sometimes we get stomach ache after eating certain food or over-eating. It can even be caused by stress, smoking, drinking alcohol, or allergies.

Whatever the cause, as long as it is short lived, there is no real problem. Use the oils in a carrier oil and massage the abdomen gently in a clockwise direction.

Oils for Stomach Ache		
Top	**Middle**	**Base**
Bergamot*	Chamomile*	Cinnamon
Peppermint*	Geranium*	
	Lavender*	
	Peppermint*	

Oils for Stomach Ache		
Top	**Middle**	**Base**
	Pine (Scotch)	
	Rosemary*	
	Sweet Fennel	

Stress

Stress is one of the most commonly referred to condition in the modern world, possibly due to the lifestyles that people now lead.

Everyone needs time to 'recharge their batteries' each day in order to maintain a calm and peaceful mindset.

Without this 'me time' eventually the body will start to show signs of stress. These signs could be headaches, not being able to sleep, being highly emotional, muscle tension or anything that is not normal to you.

Chronic stress can lead to serious conditions, including depression and dis-ease, so any stress should be treated as soon as possible to relax the body and mind.

Aromatherapy is ideal for helping you relax, and actually having the treatment in a variety of ways can be beneficial too.

Try using the oils in a warm bath, or getting a massage with them, even use them in an oil burner to scent the rooms you are working in.

Oils for Stress		
Top	**Middle**	**Base**
Basil*	Chamomile*	Benzoin
Bergamot*	Clary Sage*	Cedarwood
Clary Sage*	Cypress	Cinnamon
Grapefruit	Geranium*	Frankincense
Lemongrass	Juniper*	Jasmine*
MayChang (Litsea Cubeba)	Lavender*	Neroli*
	Melissa	Patchouli
Petitgrain	Pine (Scotch)	Rose*
Thyme*	Rosemary*	Sandalwood
		Vetiver
		Ylang Ylang

Stretch Marks

Stretch marks can happen to anyone when the skin is stretched over a short space of time, such as during pregnancy, with weight gain or even dramatic growth spurts in childhood.

They are usually visible as silvery lines although they can be purple to start with. Most stretch marks can fade over time, but aromatherapy oils can help this process.

It is a good idea to help the skin maintain its suppleness at times when stretch marks are likely to happen, such as when you are deciding to try for a baby. You can help your skin by massaging it daily with a rich oil such as Sweet Almond, Rosehip, or Cocoa Butter.

Alternatively, Bio-oil has been shown to help fade the lines and you could always add essential oils to this for additional benefit.

Oils for Stretch Marks		
Top	**Middle**	**Base**
Mandarin	Chamomile*	Frankincense
Tea Tree*	Geranium*	Myrrh
	Juniper*	Neroli*
	Lavender*	Patchouli
		Rose*
		Sandalwood

Throat Infections

Throat infections can be bacterial or viral. The most obvious symptom is a sore throat which can make it difficult to eat and drink.

It can also cause you to have enlarged tonsils and glands, a high temperature, aching muscles, a headache and even a cough and runny nose as if you have a cold or the flu.

Throat infections are common in children and young adults because they have not yet built up their immune system to fight the common bacteria and viruses that cause them.

Throat infections tend to go after 10 days and antibiotics are only needed if the infection gets very bad. If it becomes difficult to breath then seek medical attention immediately.

The best methods of using aromatherapy oils to help the soreness and infection is to use them in steam inhalations (see entry for tonsillitis for details) and in massages on the throat and neck area.

Oils for Throat Infections		
Top	**Middle**	**Base**
Clary Sage*	Clary Sage*	Ginger*
Eucalyptus*	Geranium*	
Peppermint*	Peppermint*	

Tonsillitis

Tonsillitis is an extremely sore infection of the throat and tonsils. It is very common, with most children getting it many times in their childhood.

If a child (or adult) has it many times in a year, then the decision can be made to remove their tonsils to decrease the possibility of future complications. However, contrary to popular belief, people who had had their tonsils out can still get tonsillitis, and in some cases after surgery to remove the tonsils they can grow back!

The main symptoms of tonsillitis are a severe sore throat with white pus-filled sores that can be seen on the tonsils and throat.

These can rest on the Eustachian tubes which connect the ear passages to the throat, causing earache and further pain on swallowing.

If you have tonsillitis you may also have a high temperature, headaches and in some cases, a cough.

Oils for Tonsillitis		
Top	**Middle**	**Base**
Bergamot* Eucalyptus* Tea Tree* Thyme*	Lavender*	Benzoin

Top Tip: Steam inhalations are great for tonsillitis, as is massaging the neck and throat area, coming around the ears. For addition help try using a supplement of garlic tablets and vitamin C.

Toothache

Toothache hurts!

It hurts because the pain usually comes from an irritated or exposed nerve in a tooth. Sometimes the tooth has started to decay or be infected; maybe it has broken or chipped; or maybe the tooth has come out altogether.

Gum disease can play a part too. If the gum recedes too much the nerve can be exposed this way, or infection can be allowed to get into the root of the tooth.

Whatever way the tooth has been hurt or compromised, the pain from toothache can radiate across and up the face into the temple, cheeks and forehead.

If the pain is prolonged or severe then painkillers such as ibuprofen can help. And whatever aromatherapy treatment you use, you must seek dental treatment as soon as possible.

The best method of getting rid of the pain using aromatherapy oils is to put clove oil onto the root and into the cavity. This can be done using a cotton bud with a drop of oil on it. Clove oil is not recommended for any other use than this.

Some relief can be found by using a hot compress over the cheek area. Reheat it after it cools and do not use clove oil on the face.

Oils for Toothache		
Top	**Middle**	**Base**
Cajuput

Peppermint* | Black Pepper*

Chamomile*

Peppermint* | |

Urinary Tract Infections (UTIs)

Urinary tract infections are caused by bacteria entering the urinary tract (where we 'wee' from), and are very common in women and children.

The best way to prevent a UTI is to wash your hands after using the toilet, wipe from front to back after urinating, going to the toilet and urinating after having sex and using condoms.

The symptoms can include needing to go to the loo more often but being able to pass only small amounts of urine, or not being able to go at all; pain or burning sensations on urination; pain or discomfort in the bladder; having a temperature; having cloudy or bloody urine; back, side, or kidney pain; nausea or vomiting.

Because small children can't always tell you what's going on, watch out for these additional symptoms: complaints of tummy ache; loss of appetite; not gaining weight; incontinence and bedwetting; and diarrhoea. They may cry when going to the toilet, and unable to tolerate touch to their lower abdomen.

Children with UTIs should see a medical practitioner for diagnosis and medical treatment.

Oils for Urinary Tract Infections		
Top	**Middle**	**Base**
Bergamot*	Black Pepper*	Cedarwood
Cajuput	Chamomile*	Sandalwood
Eucalyptus*	Geranium*	
Niaouli	Juniper*	
Tea Tree*	Pine (Scotch)	
Thyme*	Sweet Fennel	

Top Tip: Use a hot compress with the oils over the lower abdomen and replace when cool. Also encourage the person to drink plenty and try to ensure that drinks are not acidic or too sugary. Cranberry juice has been shown to help with bladder and urinary infections.

Vomiting

Vomiting, being sick, feeling nauseous, or queasy can happen for many reasons, from sea sickness to bad smells; illness or drug therapy; migraines to drinking too much; pregnancy to food poisoning - the list goes on.

Whatever the reason it is important to remain hydrated so try to drink little and often.

Aromatherapy can help relieve the symptoms quickly and simply.

Try inhalation on a tissue or in a room diffuser, or massage gently over the abdomen for the best results.

Oils for Vomiting		
Top	**Middle**	**Base**
Basil*	Black Pepper*	Ginger*
Bergamot*	Chamomile*	Rose*
Cajuput	Geranium*	Sandalwood
Grapefruit	Melissa	
Lemon*	Peppermint*	
Peppermint*	Sweet Fennel	

Top Tip: Ginger and Peppermint oils are excellent for reducing nausea and preventing the vomiting in the first place.

Wounds

Wounds such as cuts and grazes are very common injuries, with most causing little or no damage. You might get a scab or small scar if the skin has been broken and bleeding has occurred but mostly these will leave no mark at all.

However, deeper incisions which break the skin may cause damage to nerves, muscles, tendons and blood vessels.

These will scab and may scar both externally and internally (see scars).

Some of these deeper cuts may also require medical attention for stitching or closing using other materials.

Where there is a risk of, or actual, infection, essential oils can help to clean and treat the wound.

Oils for Wounds		
Top	**Middle**	**Base**
Bergamot*	Chamomile*	Benzoin
Eucalyptus*	Geranium*	Frankincense
Niaouli	Juniper*	Myrrh
Tea Tree*	Lavender*	Vetiver
	Rosemary*	

Top Tip: The best way to treat a wound with essential oils is to place the oils directly onto the plaster before covering the cut with it. After the plaster is no longer needed then just drip one drop of the oil directly onto the area, and continue to do this until it is completely healed. Lavender, Tea Tree, and Myrrh are potentially the best oils to use in these cases.

Wrinkles

Wrinkles are folds, ridges or creases in the skin which can be caused by numerous factors including sunlight, and smoking.

As you age the skin becomes drier, thinner and loses fat, which makes the bones and underlying structures more prominent.

As the elastin in the skin changes, the fibres no longer have the ability to go back to normal after stretching, and after time gravity can cause the skin to sag.

Although millions of pounds are spent annually on skin care, to both prevent and 'cure' wrinkles, there are some aromatherapy oils and treatments which can help.

Oils for Wrinkles		
Top	**Middle**	**Base**
Clary Sage*	Carrot Seed	Frankincense
Mandarin	Clary Sage*	Jasmine*
	Cypress	Myrrh
	Geranium*	Neroli*
	Sweet Fennel	Patchouli
		Rose*
		Sandalwood
		Ylang Ylang

Top Tip: The best method for treating wrinkles is massage using a cream or oil which is rich in texture and adding the oils to this. Massage the wrinkled area gently to encourage blood to the surface. Adding a vitamin E capsule to the cream or oil can help too.

Additionally, make sure your diet is healthy and try to give up smoking. However, ultimately prevention is better than cure, so use a high PF sun cream on your face and chest from an early age and moisturise regularly

Appendix One

Oil Compatibility Charts

Using the oil compatibility charts

The following compatibility charts will show you which essential oils can be mixed with each other. The black dots indicate a positive mix.

Take one of your essential oils and see if it is compatible with the other two on the following charts. Now check the other two.

Don't panic if they aren't all compatible.

Hopefully one of your chosen oils will be compatible with at least one of the others.

If on doubt use a cotton bud for each oil and add one drop to it. Then hold them together and waft under your nose. If you like the smell then use them together. If you don't then use different oils.

Oil Compatibility Chart A - C

	Basil	Benzoin	Bergamot	Black Pepper	Cajuput	Carrot Seed	Cedarwood	Chamomile	Cinnamon	Citronella	Clary Sage	Cypress
Basil			●	●						●	●	
Benzoin			●						●			●
Bergamot	●	●		●	●	●	●	●		●	●	●
Black Pepper	●		●									●
Cajuput			●									
Carrot Seed			●									
Cedarwood			●							●	●	●
Chamomile			●									
Cinnamon		●										
Citronella	●		●				●					
Clary Sage	●		●				●					●
Cypress		●	●	●			●				●	
Eucalyptus			●							●		
Frankincense		●		●			●		●		●	
Geranium	●		●		●		●	●			●	
Ginger									●			
Grapefruit	●		●	●			●	●	●			
Jasmine	●		●				●	●			●	
Juniper		●	●			●	●				●	●
Lavender	●	●	●		●		●	●	●		●	●
Lemon		●	●	●			●	●	●			●
Lemongrass							●			●		
Lime	●		●			●					●	

	Basil	Benzoin	Bergamot	Black Pepper	Cajuput	Carrot Seed	Cedarwood	Chamomile	Cinnamon	Citronella	Clary Sage	Cypress
Litsea Cubeba							•	•				
Mandarin			•					•				
Marjoram			•				•	•				•
Melissa			•			•	•			•		•
Myrrh	•	•										•
Neroli			•			•	•	•				
Niaouli					•							
Orange		•				•				•		•
Palmarosa			•	•				•				
Patchouli			•					•			•	
Peppermint							•					
Petitgrain		•	•			•		•				
Pine (Scotch)							•	•	•	•		
Rose		•	•		•		•	•			•	
Rosemary				•	•	•	•		•	•		
Sandalwood		•		•							•	
Spearmint	•											
Swt Fennel												
Tangerine	•							•				
Tea Tree							•			•		
Thyme			•				•	•	•			
Valerian								•				
Verbena	•		•					•				
Vetiver	•										•	
Ylang Ylang			•	•				•		•		

Oil Compatibility Chart E – L

	Eucalyptus	Frankincense	Geranium	Ginger	Grapefruit	Jasmine	Juniper	Lavender	Lemon	Lemongrass	Lime	Litsea Cubeba
Basil			●		●	●		●			●	
Benzoin		●					●	●	●			
Bergamot	●		●		●	●	●	●	●		●	
Black Pepper		●	●		●				●			
Cajuput			●					●				
Carrot Seed							●		●		●	
Cedarwood		●			●	●	●	●	●	●		●
Chamomile			●		●	●		●	●			●
Cinnamon		●		●	●			●				
Citronella	●									●		
Clary Sage		●	●			●	●	●			●	
Cypress							●	●	●			
Eucalyptus				●			●	●	●	●		●
Frankincense			●	●	●	●	●	●	●			
Geranium		●		●	●	●		●		●	●	●
Ginger	●	●	●						●		●	●
Grapefruit		●	●			●		●				●
Jasmine		●	●		●			●		●		
Juniper	●	●							●			
Lavender	●	●	●		●	●			●	●	●	
Lemon	●	●		●			●	●				
Lemongrass	●		●			●		●				
Lime			●	●				●				

	Eucalyptus	Frankincense	Geranium	Ginger	Grapefruit	Jasmine	Juniper	Lavender	Lemon	Lemongrass	Lime	Litsea Cubeba
Litsea Cubeba	●		●	●	●							
Mandarin					●	●		●	●		●	
Marjoram								●				
Melissa					●				●	●	●	
Myrrh		●	●				●	●		●		
Neroli			●			●		●	●	●	●	
Niaouli							●	●	●	●	●	
Orange		●	●	●		●	●	●				
Palmarosa			●		●	●		●		●	●	●
Patchouli		●	●	●				●		●		●
Peppermint								●				
Petitgrain			●					●				
Pine (Scotch)	●	●	●					●				
Rose			●		●	●		●		●		
Rosemary		●	●	●	●					●	●	
Sandalwood		●	●			●		●	●			
Spearmint	●					●						
Sweet Fennel	●	●	●					●	●			
Tangerine								●				
Tea Tree	●			●				●	●	●		●
Thyme							●			●		
Valerian			●					●				
Verbena			●		●			●			●	
Vetiver			●	●			●	●				
Ylang Ylang					●	●		●	●		●	●

Oil Compatibility Chart M - P

	Mandarin	Marjoram	Melissa	Myrrh	Neroli	Niaouli	Orange	Palmarosa	Patchouli	Peppermint	Petitgrain	Pine (Sctch)	Rose
Basil				•									
Benzoin				•			•				•		•
Bergamot	•	•			•			•	•		•		•
Black Pepper								•					
Cajuput							•						•
Carrot Seed			•		•		•				•		
Cedarwood		•	•		•					•	•	•	•
Chamomile	•	•			•			•	•			•	•
Cinnamon							•					•	
Citronella			•									•	
Clary Sage									•				•
Cypress		•	•	•			•				•	•	
Eucalyptus												•	
Frankincense				•			•		•			•	
Geranium				•	•		•	•	•		•	•	•
Ginger								•	•				
Grapefruit	•		•					•					•
Jasmine	•				•		•	•					•
Juniper				•		•	•						
Lavender	•	•		•	•	•	•	•	•	•	•	•	•
Lemon	•		•		•	•							•
Lemongrass			•	•	•	•		•	•				
Lime	•		•		•	•		•					•

	Mandarin	Marjoram	Melissa	Myrrh	Neroli	Niaouli	Orange	Palmarosa	Patchouli	Peppermint	Petitgrain	Pine (Sctch)	Rose
Litsea Cubeba								•	•				
Mandarin		•	•		•			•		•	•		•
Marjoram	•						•			•			
Melissa	•						•						
Myrrh								•	•				
Neroli							•	•	•		•		•
Niaouli							•				•	•	
Orange		•	•		•	•		•			•		•
Palmarosa	•			•			•				•		•
Patchouli				•	•							•	•
Peppermint	•	•			•						•		
Petitgrain	•				•		•	•					
Pine (Scotch)						•			•	•			
Rose					•		•	•	•				
Rosemary	•	•			•	•	•			•	•	•	
Sandalwood				•	•			•	•		•		•
Spearmint									•	•			
Swt Fennel		•			•								•
Tangerine		•			•			•			•		
Tea Tree	•			•			•						
Thyme	•		•		•								
Valerian				•	•		•						
Verbena					•			•					•
Vetiver		•	•				•		•				
Ylang Ylang		•			•		•	•	•		•		•

	Rose	Rosemary	Sandalwood	Spearmint	Sweet Fennel	Tangerine	Tea Tree	Thyme	valerian	Verbena	Vetiver	Ylang Ylang
Basil				●		●				●	●	
Benzoin	●		●									
Bergamot	●									●		●
Black Pepper		●	●									●
Cajuput	●							●				
Carrot Seed		●								●		
Cedarwood	●	●					●					
Chamomile	●					●			●	●		●
Cinnamon		●						●				
Citronella		●					●					●
Clary Sage	●		●								●	
Cypress		●	●				●					
Eucalyptus				●	●		●					
Frankincense		●	●		●							
Geranium	●	●	●		●				●	●	●	
Ginger		●					●				●	
Grapefruit	●	●								●		●
Jasmine	●		●	●							●	●
Juniper												
Lavender	●		●		●	●	●	●	●	●	●	●
Lemon	●		●		●		●					●
Lemongrass		●					●					
Lime	●	●								●		●

	Rose	Rosemary	Sandalwood	Spearmint	Sweet Fennel	Tangerine	Tea Tree	Thyme	valerian	Verbena	Vetiver	Ylang Ylang
Litsea Cubeba							•					•
Mandarin	•	•					•					
Marjoram		•				•					•	•
Melissa					•						•	
Myrrh			•				•		•			
Neroli	•	•	•			•			•	•		•
Niaouli		•			•							
Orange	•	•					•		•		•	•
Palmarosa	•		•			•				•		•
Patchouli	•		•	•							•	•
Peppermint		•		•								
Petitgrain		•	•			•						•
Pine (Scotch)		•										
Rose			•		•					•		•
Rosemary				•	•		•			•		
Sandalwood	•				•						•	•
Spearmint		•				•	•				•	
Sweet Fennel	•	•	•						•			
Tangerine				•								
Tea Tree		•		•								
Thyme		•					•					
Valerian												•
Verbena	•	•										•
Vetiver			•	•								
Ylang Ylang	•		•						•	•		

Appendix Two

Oil Mixing Sheets

Oil Mixing Sheet

Name:

Age:

Do not use any oil on a child under 16 unless a qualified Aromatherapist has been consulted, or you are confident in your abilities.

Do you or your client have any of the following conditions?

Diabetes☐

Pregnancy☐

Sensitive Skin☐

Breast Feeding☐

Hypertension / High Blood Pressure☐

Epilepsy☐

If any of the above are checked please refer to the list of oils outlined on page nine, which are not to be used, and delete any of these from your list below.

Top (2 drops)	**Middle** (7 Drops)	**Base** (1 drop)

Oils to use:

Carrier Oil used:

Oils to avoid due to adverse reaction:

Please photocopy this blank form as required.

Note	Condition			Note	Condition			Note	Condition		
Top	1	2	3	**Middle**	1	2	3	**Base**	1	2	3
Basil				Black Pepper				Benzoin			
Bergamot				Carrot Seed				Cedarwood			
Cajuput				Chamomile				Cinnamon			
Clary Sage				Clary Sage				Frankincense			
Eucalyptus				Cypress				Ginger			
Grapefruit				Geranium				Jasmine			
Lemon				Juniper				Myrrh			
Lime				Lavender				Neroli			
Lemongrass				Marjoram				Patchouli			
Litsea cubeba				Melissa				Rose			
Mandarin				Peppermint				Sandalwood			
Niaouli				Pine (Scotch)				Valerian			
Orange				Rosemary				Vetiver			
Peppermint				Sweet Fennel				Ylang Ylang			
Petitgrain											
Tea Tree											
Thyme											
Verbena											

Please photocopy as necessary

Adverse Side Effects

If you, or the person you have mixed for, use any oil and have an adverse side effect please list those oils used here and detail the reaction that happened.

Name:

Top	Middle	Base	Carrier	Reaction

Conduct a sensitivity test for each oil and note reaction.

Oil	Reaction

Once reaction is known this oil should not be used by this person again.

Use a separate sheet for each person

Appendix Three

Purchasing and storing your essential oils

How to purchase your essential oils.

Always buy essential oils from a reputable company, or one that has been recommended. Try not to buy from market stalls at your local market unless you know exactly where the oils have been produced from. Good sellers will always have the country of origin marked on their bottles, and will have good information on them, such as the ingredients, and percentages if appropriate.

Do not buy perfume oils as these as not the same as essential oils and will not have the same effect.

Make sure that the oil you are buying is not adulterated with something else unless it is an expensive oil such as Rose or Jasmine. Some oils will be diluted in a carrier oil and this should be mentioned on the label. Only the really expensive ones should do this, so if you see Lavender or Tea Tree in a carrier oil then avoid it as it is less expensive to buy the pure oils and mix them yourself.

Oils can be expensive as it takes so much of them to produce one drop, so shop around and make sure that you are comparing like for like.

Always check the ingredients, and if they do not say the oil is made only from natural ingredients or essential oils then you can be sure that they will contain synthetic products or fragrance oils. If it says 'made with essential oils', then it will contain something else as well. These extra ingredients or dilution will not help in any way.

The quality and price will be affected by a number of different factors, such as how rare the plant it is made from is (It takes tonnes of roses to make one ounce of oil), which country it grows in and comes from, what growing conditions it needs (does it take years for the plant to grow to a state where the oil can be extracted? If so it will be more expensive), what standards the distiller have and how much oil can be extracted from each plant (see comment about Roses above!)

Therefore, the price and quality can vary immensely.

Look where they are stored in a shop and avoid oils that have been stored near a window as light will deteriorate the effect. Also check the expiration date and only go for ones that have a long shelf life left.

How to store your essential oils.

Essential oils should be stored in blue or amber glass bottles in a cool dark place, with a plastic dropper rather than a rubber stopper / dropper as this will disintegrate over time and could contaminate the oils

Recommended Reading

If you are interested in aromatherapy and want to build up your library, I recommend the following books which have helped me throughout the years:

The Directory of Essential Oils, Wanda Sellar; The C. W. Daniel Co Ltd

The Fragrant Pharmacy, Valerie Anne Worwood; Macmillian

The Complete Book of Essential Oils and Aromatherapy, Valerie Worwood, New World Library

Practical Aromatherapy, Penny Rich; Parragon

The Very Essence; Lisa Burke, Phillilp Chambers, Simon Mallinson; Likisma Presentations Ltd.

Aromatherapy in Essence; Chrissie Wildwood; Masada Ltd.

The Encyclopaedia of Essential Oils, Julia Lawless, Element Books Ltd.

Aromatherapy for Women, Maggie Tisserand; Thorsons Publishing Group

Aromatherapy: an A-Z, Patricia Davies, The C.W. Daniel Co Ltd.

About the Author

Kath Hoskisson-Craven is a qualified Complementary Therapist with 20 years' experience of practicing Aromatherapy, Reflexology, and Indian Head Massage as well as other treatments. She taught complementary therapies at Halesowen College and wrote the first Foot Massage Level One course for the awarding body ONC.

Her interest in aromatherapy started at a young age using Lavender and Tea Tree oils during her childhood and teenage years and moving on to more advanced use during her early twenties.

Kath is now using herbs in combination with oils to make healing lotions and bars, and enjoys foraging for these herbs in the local woods and fields where she lives. She shares her times between working as a Forest School Lead; doing her complementary therapies; and being with her two children, husband, dog, cat and three chickens.

I'd love to hear about your successes and experiences with this book. You can post them on my Facebook page where you can also learn more about herbs and oils, recipes and tips for a healthier natural lifestyle. facebook.com/thepurplehealingroom.

Did you enjoy this book?
Please leave me a review on Amazon as I'd love to hear your thoughts about it.